Other titles by

John P Gibson

TOUT

LISA'S

The Algarve Story

Kamauna 2908

Any of these books can be purchased at;
http://www.lulu.com/spotlight/johnpgibson

Dead Next Tuesday

www.heddonpublishing.com

"SO SIMPLE, WHO KNEW?"

"The perceived challenge of becoming, and staying healthy."

A BOOK
BY
JOHN P. GIBSON

INTRODUCTION

John Gibson makes his home in Cobble Hill, BC Canada on the East coast of Vancouver Island. He has authored many articles in newsletters and other publications through his websites. He has been an activist for the natural way of healing the body and of course our planet.

"So Simple, Who Knew?" is his first book on the topic of healing through a natural process as opposed to the synthetic system we are all too familiar with. In this book he tries to convey to you the reader the problems we face globally and the actions we can, and should take to eradicate them.

This is more a book on fixing the planet, and in turn that will ultimately fix us. The human element to the equation. John hopes to start something within the individual to make changes that need to be made to bring this planet, and we as humans to a state of harmony and balance.

John's future works will likely be in the fiction genre as that is what he very much enjoys writing. He thought he should however unburden himself first with this book. There is no certainty that there will not be a follow-up to this book, it will be a wait and see what happens situation.

If you wish to communicate with John directly you can send an email to this address: johnpgibson@writeme.com

DISCLAIMER

All information within this book is for the soul purpose of education. Any application of a lifestyle change should only be considered with the guidance of ones health care professional. The information expressed by the author is of his opinion and his opinion only and not to be used for the diagnosis, or treatment of any health issue. It is not an expressed opinion of any person or persons in any professional field expressed or inferred in this book.

FORWARD

"A little good food, a little movement, a little stress free life, some quality rest. These are all that are required for a healthy life."

Now that you know how simple it is, you can put the book down and live a good life, or maybe find some enjoyment in reading through every chapter and possibly learn something new. I hope you enjoy the read.

Health has become a passion of mine, and as you will soon find out, I become very vocal about many things we as humans are doing to our home, this planet, Earth, that indirectly or directly is affecting our health and that of many other species.

I have spent more than twenty years exploring the ever increasing complexities of getting and staying healthy. As this book starts out, you can see that living a healthy life is far from complicated. Complication is something we humans seem to thrive on, why, I do not know. Through the years I have tried many systems only to find out later they had many flaws. I then discarded them. This happened many times, and I assume will continue as I have an insatiable appetite for information..especially when it comes to living a healthy lifestyle.

As I march on through the years approaching the ultimate goal of life itself, the end. I cannot help but notice how many older people can live a reasonably healthy lifestyle doing almost all of the wrong things. This is where I now believe that we as humans must keep it simple, as these people have done for an entire lifetime, we have to keep it simple, or the complications we so readily create will be our ultimate undoing.

As you read through the chapters, I often repeat certain points. I do this because they represent something more important, and repetition is what anchors new process's into our sub conscious. I too also seem to get into certain rants about other subjects, this is just me and I am using this medium as a vent. I certainly do not want you to take it too seriously, and it is certainly not my intention to offend anyone, we must keep the stress to a minimum.

In some ways this book is more about realizing the damage we have done to our planet and why it is we have to start the repair process. We as a species have to realize we are an integral part of the process of nature, and to try and break away from that, have caused the problems we are facing today.

If in anyway this information can help you or friends or family, then what I set out to do has been achieved. I wish you the reader, a wonderful and healthy life. Just make sure to throw a little adventure into it, and don't take anything too seriously, and do your best not to use plastic bags.

John P. Gibson
March 2011

CONTENTS

MY STORY

I am not a Doctor nor a scientist. I am not a politician or an academic. What I am is just a regular run of the mill Canadian citizen who has tried for most of his life to do all of the right things hopefully at the right times.

Foremost is my dedication to improving my personal health and the health of those around me, and the health of our planet we all call home. I have spent the past 20 years working on educating myself about the best ways to achieve this and live a healthy life. Almost to the point of being obsessive about it...so some of my family and friends have noted on more than a few occasions.

Over the years I have improved in health considerably through the dedicated actions of proper nutrition, regular exercise, and stress reduction. At the age of 33, I started my quest for better health due entirely to a problem with my knees. The tendons connecting the knee caps had worn out on both.

Too much activity when I was younger, combined with a poor diet and lack of knowledge about proper warm up exercises, and the role that nutrition played in the maintenance and repair of damaged tissue. I was at this time also eating a very poor diet with the consumption of far too many meats, bad fats, alcohol, and simple sugars.

My specialist informed me I had a condition they called "Jumpers Knee". I had been active in school sports, namely track and field where I was constantly jumping or sprinting. Along with snow skiing, water skiing, ice skating, soccer, and just general running around, as a boy usually does.

I, not knowing, was wearing out my tendons to the point where my specialist informed me, at the nice old age of 33 that I should stop running, skating, hiking, baseball, and anything else that aggravated my condition. Or deal with the consequences, one, being on pain killers or last resort if worn out tendons detached...to have an operation to re-attach them.

He also informed me that my condition would never improve and I should accept the fact that I now had the knees of a 70 year old. And believe me, they felt like it, especially after a game of baseball, one of my favourite pastimes.

My knees would hurt so bad it could take up to three or four days for the pain to subside, just in time for the next baseball game. I would try over the counter pain killers, to no avail. I quickly stopped using them as they affected me in other ways. All I could do was live with the pain.

I was however, not prepared to hang up my baseball cleats just yet. I began to do some research on my own about exercise and diet and came across an article, about the effects of consuming red meats, especially today's commercially produced beef, and how it relates to damaging effects on joint ligaments, cartilage, and tendons. I decided at that moment to try an experiment. As I was a big fan of meat, any kind of meat, I would abstain from eating any meat of any kind for one month to see if there was any validity to the report I had just read.

Remarkably, within three weeks my knees started to improve, this prompted me to delve further into research and apply proper exercise to the formula. I quickly signed up at the local gym and started on a strict exercise program. Again, another great improvement on my knees.

Of course along with my knees feeling better, many other parts of me were also feeling much better. It has now been more than 20 years of regular dietary and exercise programs and my health in general has been very good. My knees were in great shape, and I could not remember a time when I had felt so healthy. Life it seemed was back in my control. However, things would change, drastically for the worse.

It was early in 2004 that I began to have what I considered some major health concerns. I was unable to work efficiently at a local construction job I had, and was confused as to what it was that was happening to my body that I had worked so hard at keeping fit and in great running order. Now, again, not being part of the majority when it comes to believing exactly everything that my doctor has to say about any condition I might have, I always question the cause of the symptoms.

This often gets me some strange reactions, strange looks, or heated rebuttals. I have never found myself hard to get along with, but sometimes talking with professionals that are supposed to know what should be done in almost any circumstance, I find it strange to say the least to just arbitrarily attach a condition to a symptom, or symptoms, without proper testing. I sometimes feel as if they (The Professionals) (Doctors) think I am not telling them the truth.

Now where is all this leading to you ask? Let me elaborate more about the symptoms I was experiencing. Some of you reading this will be able to relate, others I'm sure will think that I am just plain crazy. (We'll talk about that later).

Here are some of the symptoms that I experienced. Some came on gradually over a two to three year period, most however came on suddenly. Within a two to three week time frame.

Here goes then, SYMPTOMS; "Hot flashes, clammy hands, chest pains, (on and off), ringing in both ears, headaches, foggy brain, (look it up on the internet), aches and pains in neck and shoulders, elevated heart rate, shortness of breath, high blood pressure, digestive problems, forgetfulness, always fatigued, poor co-ordination, bad breath, excessive body odour, bleeding gum's, soreness in jaw, poor sleep, lack of taste and smell, never feeling hungry, dryness in mouth, bad temper, and an elevated artistic ability. (Strange, yes...but true.)

There were other symptoms that would come and go as well. Apart from the ringing in my ears and the bleeding gum's, which started about three years previously, still, probably brought on by the same cause, the remainder of the symptoms manifested rather quickly. All of this happening to a very fit and healthy person. So I thought. I had regular testing done through my doctor and all the test results came back with flying colours according to my doctor. I was a normal, healthy male of 49 years.

Normal that is with a lot of symptoms I could not explain, or my doctor for that matter. My doctor was not willing to investigate any further...my ten minutes were up. Her response was for me to see a psychiatrist, consider that it might be depression, and if they, (the psychiatrist's) believed it to be depression, then to start me on antidepressants...(DRUGS! We all know how well they work on a long term basis). Well, if I didn't think it was depression that was the cause of my symptoms, I certainly wasn't feeling all that positive now. In fact who wouldn't feel depressed with all of those symptoms.

As someone who really likes to be sure of things, I thought a suggestion to my doctor was in order, that maybe we should do more testing, like maybe for heavy metal toxicity.(Toxaemia). I thought this was a reasonable course of action as I had over the years worked in the construction trade and other jobs that had put me in close proximity with deadly chemicals where I'm sure I had been exposed to all kinds of deadly substances with a less than desirable reputation.

Well..,I guess I should know better than to one-up my doctor. My doctor after hearing this let out a series of laughs and then said to me under no uncertain terms that this was not going to happen and that I should not even venture there. I was confused, to say the least, and not just from my ongoing symptoms. Was not my doctor supposed to find underlying problems that are affecting her patients health and proceed to look for answers to a solution?

Apparently not. I got the impression that this was an easy way out for her, as many thousands of people are diagnosed with depression and are promptly administered antidepressants. (Which have been proven for the most part to be ineffectual.) Did my doctor not take an oath..."First do no harm." Had she been influenced to cut costs for our Government, health care plan, or by the large drug companies to take the easy way out and put large profits ahead of ethical and honest behaviour. I mean really...if you have all of the symptoms that I had, wouldn't you be depressed too?

I refused to believe it was depression only, and now I had to look elsewhere for answers.. It was apparent that our   relationship was out the door, and so was I to look for a new doctor and hopefully answers to the underlying cause of all my symptoms.

CHAPTER ONE - "TODAY'S REALITY"

Have you ever been feeling a little under the weather? Maybe not quite as chipper as you are usually? Has this been happening for an extended period of time? Happening more often? Do you know several others that complain of similar symptoms? Is it common place to compete with one another around the water cooler to see who has the worst cough, or cold, or flu? Welcome to the 21st century.

These days it is hard to find anyone that is in an average state of health let alone a superior state, or even a state that would be considered normal by natures standards. Our planet is in deep trouble, too many people, too much pollution, and far too many man-made chemicals, more than 70,000 of them, and many of them we ingest intentionally or unintentionally through the air we breath, water we drink, or food we consume, even some of the clothes we wear. Is it any wonder so many are so sick.

A main contributor to our health, or lack of it are the toxins we put into our bodies everyday, most through what we eat. Many more get into our bodies when we agree to use highly toxic drugs...or as medical personnel refer to as prescription medication. Almost every man-made drug has some sort of side effect that in some cases is often worse than the disease itself.

Our water supply on this planet is contaminated. Some experts believe there is not a drop of surface water that is not. Our municipal water systems are continually bombarded with toxic chemicals just to make it safe for us to consume, and even then it is far from safe. I always drink filtered or distilled water. Not even bottled water is safe, not to mention the incredible numbers of plastic water bottles that end up in ever growing landfills, or as we use to call them...garbage dumps, or the massive sections of ocean where garbage finds its way. The Pacific Ocean has its own garbage patch the size of Texas. Mostly plastics!

With millions of cars driving the highways everyday our air quality is diminishing rapidly.

The actual percentage of oxygen is getting less as the centuries march on. No wonder, with all the deforestation we create every year.

Mostly just to raise crops for cattle or to make space to raise cattle itself. Our sick care programs, (I call them sick care for the simple reason there are no more healthy people around.) are busting at the seams financially and to find reasonable care one must look outside the system and pay much more for it.

More than 50 years ago we were told by experts that we had better clean up our act or suffer dire consequences. To this day we have not heeded those words. Our planet is in worse shape and our health is the worst it has ever been. Even our children as young as two or three are being medicated. Where am I going with all of this doom and gloom?

I just want it to be clear to you the reader that we have poisoned our nest and other than a few small organizations, no one is doing anything to clean it up. So what do we do? And what does this have to do with your health? Everything.

Most disease's can be traced back to environmental circumstances, mostly man-made toxins that co-exist with all of us everyday of our lives. Toxins can enter our bodies through many entry points. Breathing, skin, food, water, medications, the list goes on.

With me it was an accumulation of many toxins over many years, which brings us to a point. Are we all not absorbing toxins? Over many years? I believe many of the disease's today can be traced to toxins we have exposed our bodies to over many years, even while we were in our mothers womb.

It is far too often people hear the words, "We don't know how people contract this disease." Maybe we should clean up our planet and my guess is a lot of our health issues will be cleaned up as well. So how do we avoid these toxins? Bad news my friend...right now we can't. Like I said earlier, there are over 70,000 of them and more being produced all the time. These toxins are in us all and will one day cause us some kind of problems. We can however do some preventive maintenance and do everything in our power to ensure future generations are free from this mess we have created for hundreds or perhaps thousands of years.

What I hope to achieve throughout the rest of this book is a plan of action for you and others to rid yourself of these toxins to the best of your ability. These toxins can cause so much grief, and to plan out a lifestyle that is in balance with our planet and our personal health.

Many will disagree with the information I will share, others will try it and more than likely experience positive results from it. The formula is simple, and has been the same for many thousands of years. "Live with, and contribute to the benefit of Nature". By doing this we all will become healthier and an asset to our home. "Earth".

By following certain sets of rules we can make this planet what it once was, and instead of hundreds of thousands of species going extinct, we can see new ones evolving to make an abundance of resources not only for us but for all other living organisms on this planet for many thousands of years to come. Sound a bit too big for you? I understand. But how about just dealing with you? If you, make some small changes right now, do you think that would have an impact?

Well my guess is it would take many of us, but it still starts with you. By making some simple but yet effective choices you will become healthier and the side effects will be the repair of our planet. Sounds like a pretty good trade off to me.

In the following chapters I will get into detail about what it is everyone needs to do in order to be, and stay, healthy. This in turn helps to clean up our planet and ensure many more species will remain healthy, which is exactly what our planet needs right now and in the future. I'm not saying you have to give up anything, just make better decisions with the lifestyle you have chosen.

This is not about losing weight...unless you want to, not about giving up certain foods...unless you want to, not about becoming a radical...unless you want to. But we do have to make changes in the everyday things that we do, and we have to make sure future generations understand how important it is to do so, or they may not have a user friendly planet to call their home. If we do not clean up our home and treat it with the respect it deserves we as humans will without a doubt become extinct and take many other species with us.

What a shame, we as humans have been given so many talents and the capacity to improve almost anything to make life better for all. Sure, a few seem to have everything they ever wanted, but are they truly living a good life? Is the pursuit of power and money really necessary? Balance is the key. In all things, balance is number one.

I am extending to you a challenge. One, to at least read through this book. I know some of you may not agree with what I have to say...I understand that. But to really get it, you must explore any and all points of view and possibilities. And two, make a positive change in your daily life, no matter how small. One simple change for the better.

So if you do want to become healthier, lose weight, quit smoking, eat better, feel better, think better...then read on, maybe some of this will make sense to you. It did to me, but only after I applied the information and took action. Before we get started in chapter two, there are a few things you will have to do. First, start today with an open mind. Listen and read and make no judgements.

Try things, and give it enough time to take effect. Do not be too hard on yourself, that's not what it's about. I will give you resources for getting answers from me either by website, email, or webinars at the end of the book. Feel free to experiment a little, we are all different and no one system is ideal for everyone. You may even develop something that could be beneficial to many others, anything is possible.

You are probably asking how is it you can save the planet just by being healthier? Well it's not likely you can do it all on your own, you will need some help from others. The more the merrier. By making sound, responsible, lifestyle choices you can't help but improve your health, the health of the planet, and the health of others close to you. For example, walking five miles everyday and incorporating that walk into doing daily chores saves you wear and tear on the car and savings in fuel costs. You become healthier and the planet does because you use less fuel and emit fewer toxins into the air. Simple.

Just one positive thing you decide to do, and the planet is on its way to being healthier, and over time, more, clean, toxic free oxygen for you and others to breath. Every chapter is devoted to one part of the formula. I will go into detail about the importance of it, the positive results you get, and the positive results the planet gets. So lets get with the program.

CHAPTER TWO - "GETTING RID OF TOXINS"

As I have said before, there are more than 70,000 man made chemicals on this planet, I will bring this up other times throughout this book because of its importance to our survival and health, or, our decline and sickness. Most are harmful to both you and the planet. Why? It takes thousands of years for Eco systems to adjust to new stimuli...especially a species like us. Most toxins that enter our system, as well as the planet we live on, create havoc.

Our systems do not recognize the new substance and try to eliminate it. If it cannot eliminate it, the substance usually gets stored somewhere in our bodies, usually in fatty areas like the liver, heart, digestive system, and brain. Just like us the planet must do the same thing. It must find a way to deal with the toxin. It may be stored in our water supply, the earth we grow our food in, and even the air we breath.

As I expressed earlier I went through a troubling time with a host of symptoms that my regular doctor had no answers for. After seeing a qualified doctor who administered a multitude of tests including really getting to know me and my medical history. This is what he found. The envelope please.

I had elevated amounts of Arsenic and Mercury in my system, a couple of deadly toxins that are in some amounts present in nature, but generally small enough amounts when introduced into our bodies it can be handled by our immune system. With ever increasing man-made accumulations of Mercury and Arsenic, my body, even as healthy as it was, (So I thought) did not stand a chance against these two formidable deadly toxins.

Mercury is everywhere in small amounts. In our food, air, and water. Arsenic is also prevalent in small amounts. Add in the mercury used in industry (Processing of coal is one), the use of mercury fillings for cavities, mercury in the production of cement, black and white photo processing, my body didn't stand a chance. (I had been involved in all of these industries).

If you have ever heard of **"The Mad Hatter Disease"** It was exactly what I was going through. Mad Hatters were called just that because they worked with mercury in the processing of felt for hats back in the 1800's. They did not live too long and went completely crazy as well as exhibiting many of the symptoms I described earlier with my own illness.

That's because mercury just loves to mess around with your brain, which explains all of the other symptoms. I won't go into great detail about this horrible disease, you can Google it on the internet and find loads of information. But I do have to point out that many people today exhibit signs of the "Mad Hatter" disease.

My "qualified" doctor had me go on a strict diet to help purge my system of these harsh toxins and recommended I have my fillings replaced with non toxic ones. Most people, especially of my generation have these Amalgam fillings. He suggested I not even think about having them replaced until my body was strong enough for the procedure. Six months later after being on a strict cleansing diet he said I was fit enough to have them replaced in two stages so as not to create more problems with any excess mercury that might re-enter the body during the procedure.

Within three weeks of having the last of the mercury removed from my mouth, I felt like a new person. I had the fillings replaced in two separate procedures spread over about four months. To this day I still incorporate parts of the diet and vitamin protocol to assist in the ongoing effort to eliminate toxins from my body.

Now, I was an extreme case. My doctor informed me that my system was shutting down. Liver, heart, kidneys were all being stressed and without intervention I may have had only a year or two to live. I know, scary stuff. Now, most people have mild symptoms that are more than likely a result of a toxic overload, but most doctors are too quick to place a label on the symptoms and prescribe drugs to reduce the affects of the symptoms, not even addressing the underlying problem that causes the symptoms. I still must be careful when I am around certain toxic environments.

My body is now very sensitive to a wide range of chemicals, even some in perfumes and cosmetics. The chemical properties of many solvents, paints, and industrial cleaning agents cause me even more grief. When your Doctor prescribes drugs for symptoms you are having, he is only adding to the toxic overload to your system.

Sure it feels better now, but a bottle of wine, case of beer, or smoking a marijuana cigarette would accomplish the same thing. Not that I am suggesting this course of action, they are all damaging to the body if abused. We are just to eager to follow along a path of destruction that could just be worse than the initial problem.

The more sensible approach is to get a detailed history of the patient to find out if the patient has been in contact with any abnormal amounts of any toxins. Through diet, profession, hobby, proximity to large industrial sites, (working or shut down). In many cases it is in the diet and an easy fix. Just stop eating the poisonous foods. But too many patients aren't informed this way.

I often get the response when I suggest a change in diet, "Well, they haven't proven that eating large amounts of saturated fats is bad for you." But they are not willing to prove me or any of the experts wrong, which would mean a change in diet for no less than six months to a year, and possibly for the rest of ones life. Example...type I and II Diabetes.

To rid the body totally of toxins these days is probably unrealistic. We are continually bombarded with toxins 24 hours a day, every day of our lives. We need to adopt a daily regime of toxic purging with a more focused plan three to four times per year. I would suggest the lemonade cleanse, or Master Cleanse as it is called. It not only allows your body some down time to regenerate, but also allows toxins to leave through your waste systems.

Think of it like owning a car. Most people take it in for a regular check up, maybe every two to three months. Oil change, fluid checks, check tires, brakes, transmission, belts, and more. Most would never think of not doing this important servicing. So why don't we do it to our bodies? A much more sophisticated and highly technical piece of hardware. By flushing out our system we get rid of nasty toxins that have built up in our digestive system sometimes for decades.

These stores of old decaying fecal matter release toxins into our system over and over again. When this old fecal matter is removed through fasting and flushing, our body has the opportunity to regenerate new and healthier cells to do the millions of chores necessary to maintain a healthy body.

In some cases there can be more than ten pounds of this decaying, putrefying fecal matter lining our intestines. Just by doing a short cleanse with a proper flush, you could not only drop an easy ten pounds right there, but also feel so much better. By removing these deadly toxins our bodies now have a chance to become healthier. The first place you notice this is your skin. It starts to look smoother and has more colour to it. It works much more efficiently, I am talking about your skin, (Your largest organ) will now help to eliminate toxins much more easily.

If you are prone to body aches and pains, they tend to dissipate, you have more energy, your bowel movements are more regular and of proper consistency, your eyes look better, your hair softer, and your organs work so much better. Your heart especially, bringing it into a range that is healthy and productive.

Another obvious place to eliminate toxins even before they enter our bodies is to make sure they don't enter our homes or bodies in the first place. A good book to read is **"Detoxify Or Die"** *Sherry A Rogers*.

She identifies many toxins that are present in our

homes, especially plastics. Plastics are a difficult one to eliminate completely but we can reduce and use only plastics that are food safe, or use glass instead. Our carpets, paint, insulation, TV's, computers, cookware, microwaves, heating systems, the list goes on. All of these things can contribute to a very toxic home. Again, it is difficult to eliminate all unless you are building from scratch. We truly do have to become more aware of what we purchase and how we live. Some experts believe that a new born child already has many of the toxins in there bodies that took a lifetime for our grandparents to accumulate.

Plastics are used everywhere, even in our cars where a lot of us spend a lot of our time, and some time with our young children. We just need to be more diligent when it comes to purchasing things in plastic, or are made of plastic. When shopping for groceries do your best to buy things that aren't packaged in plastic. Opt for glass or paper or cans. If you can't avoid purchasing items that are packaged heavily with plastic, take the time to remove your product from the excessive packaging and leave the packaging at the store.

If more of us did this, the stores would then send

all of this packaging back to the supplier, who would then in turn send it back to the manufacturer, who would then in turn send it back to the plastic manufacturer, who would then have to come up with a better idea on how to package it. It seems simple, not likely to happen, but when it comes to making a profit, most companies put our health, and the health of our planet on the back burner.

I have noticed that some manufacturers are now asking that any of their products that are to be returned for refund must be returned with original packaging. Now they want us to store this toxic stuff in our homes for who knows how long. Driving less also helps with the toxins being released into our atmosphere. Try and plan your trips so that you can get more done in one day and leave the car sitting at home more often. If you live close to a supermarket or mall where you do most of your shopping, pick a nice day and walk to get your groceries, bring the children to help, treat it as an exercise day.

You will do yourself a favour, and the planet. Reducing the number of trips you make in your vehicle cuts down not only on pollution, but saves you money on the fuel savings, and makes for a healthier you. Better all the way around. Another great way to reduce toxins from entering into the system is to put your dry goods right after a shopping day into glass containers, then dispose of the plastic wrapping or bags they had been stored in. This way you are sure that the plastics won't leech anymore toxins into the food that you will consume.

Water. I will get into this one in more detail in a later chapter, but for now here are a couple of ideas to help out. If you can, get a small water distiller. **(WaterWise)** has a great counter top model. It takes a bit of work, but you will be sure that the water you consume is not contaminated. Bottled water is a no-no! Not only does it cost too much. (Nearly twice the cost to produce it than it costs to buy.) But then you have to get rid of the plastic bottles when you are finished with them, and in most cases the water in those bottles is worse than your tap water!

For a small family that consumes a normal amount of water per day, you save money by filtering it yourself and storing it ideally in glass containers in the fridge. Next best, charcoal filters in-line or carafes. The planet will thank you for this too, less garbage to deal with. It takes thousands of years for plastic to completely decompose. And once it is back into the environment, who knows what happens? Again with the plastics, when shopping for your children, whether it be clothing or toys, be mindful of what the products are made of.

Sure, it's nice to recycle plastic, but into clothing? Our bodies are very efficient at absorbing almost anything. So if plastic leeches chemicals and we wear plastic, it's only safe to say that our bodies will absorb some of the chemicals. Just like smothering our skin with creams, make-up, sunscreen, and insect repellents. We have to get smart about what we come into contact with, even airborne chemicals can enter our bodies through our skin.

A very serious group of toxins include the family of insecticides. Including pesticides, fungicides, fertilizers and any other man-made chemical to enhance the production of flowers, vegetables, fruits, and grains. Most store bought flowers and plants have been grown with large amounts of these toxins, it's no wonder so many people now have allergies. When purchasing fruit and vegetables, it is best to get them from a local source and one that practices organic farming. Always wash vegetables and fruit thoroughly before consuming.

Certain profession's run a risk of being in contact with harmful toxins. Be aware of these potential hazards and wear proper safety gear. Or better yet, get into a profession that does not harm you. It would be a real challenge to find a profession these days that does not have some kind of toxic problem. Even as I write this book in front of a computer, I am being bombarded with many toxins from the leeching of chemicals from the plastic, or the breathing in of small amounts of mercury, even the electrical output has an effect.

To eliminate all toxins from entering our bodies would be nearly impossible. But we can do a lot to reduce the numbers as I have explained. I will get into this in a more in depth way in future chapters. When presented with the alternatives, it can seem far too overwhelming to make all the changes necessary.

All you need to do is make a start in the right

direction and just do one thing to start. As you get better at replacing old habits with new ones, the shift will be considerably easier and faster. The first step is to get a qualified diagnosis of YOU! From a qualified Doctor. If you have no problems I would suggest getting ready for a cleanse. I mentioned earlier that this was a large part of my program to become healthy once again.

There are two cleanses I recommend. First the **RESET PROGRAM** through **USANA Health Sciences**. A great tasting easy to incorporate 5 day cleanse. I will elaborate on this one in a later chapter. Once you are on track with your diet and exercise the 10 day **Lemonade Master Cleanse** an excellent way to rejuvenate your system and get rid of a lot of the toxins and excess accumulation in your intestines.

This one you can get information on the internet. Just do a search for Lemonade Cleanse or Master Cleanse and be sure to read all the pros and cons before attempting this cleanse. It does take some preparation and a strong will to complete, but it is well worth it. You will feel almost brand new again. Skin looks and feels better, you will sleep better, heart rate is better, stress levels down, digestive system rejuvenated, better colour in your eyes, hair is better, and your brain functions better. Not to mention the savings in food costs for ten days.

These cleanse' should be done at the start of your program so when you re-introduce food to your diet your system can start fresh with proper nutrients and quality food. Now I'm not going to say you have to become a vegan, or eat fish only, but I will help you figure out a meal plan that works for you and your family. I like my chocolate too. But it is important to understand why we get hungry, and what we should be consuming for the best health results. So, for you red meat eaters, the ones that like to have some red meat every meal and then some, you are going to have to make a real shift away from this meat.

If you really like it, then set a long term goal to consume it only once or twice per week, ideally, less is better. And for some people, never again. I haven't eaten red meat for over 20 years now...I'm still here. I do believe that some people should consume a little red meat, and I will elaborate on this later in the book.

Food combining can be another great way to get rid of toxins and get your health back in line. I have done extensive research on the author and activist **Dr. Herbert M. Shelton** and agree with most of his writings. I would like to quote one of his paragraphs from his book;

(Food Combining Made Easy). *"That haphazard eaters may learn to combine their foods by rules that are based on the Physiology of digestion, foul stools, gas and discomfort that accompany conventional eating, is a fact that any doubter may discover for himself by giving the matter a fair test. Any medical man who will give it a test may discover this for himself.*

That medical men pretend that they are "scientific" and are wedded to the "scientific method" while refusing to put the matter to a test is an evidence of their prejudice and bigotry. They reject the "scientific method" if and when
there is reason to think that the results of a test may disturb the customs of the people and practices of the profession. The test might show them to be wrong."

Our main focus here is to educate ourselves about how and why we eat. If it was just a case of eating what we liked for the sake of enjoyment, and we could thrive and maintain excellent health on this kind of diet, I would purchase and consume nothing else but chocolate, wine, and French fries. Ah, but that is not the case. We must eat certain foods at certain times. So if this is true, would it not be prudent to eat the best available foods for our health and to eat them at the proper times?

If you truly care about how you want to live your life so that you are physically capable and mentally capable of doing the things you enjoyed doing when you were a teenager, well into your eighties and beyond, then you will have to adopt a different set of rules on how, and when you consume the right kinds of good quality foods. The planet will also benefit by your new choices. People are notorious for complicating things to a point where no one can understand it, or wants to. Maintaining excellent health and a proper body weight, and fixing our planet, is not rocket science.

The formula is very simple; Proper diet + Moderate exercise + Quality rest + Low stress = EXCELLENT HEALTH! I often hear from many people, "I have tried everything and I can't seem to lose any weight!" or "I'm on this diet and all I can lose is five pounds, then I always put it back on." There are many more, but this gives you an idea.

The problem is, humans are lazy. They don't want to exercise, diet, or do almost anything else required to become healthier. If you are not willing to step out of your comfort zone on a continual basis, you will never achieve any lofty goals you have set for yourself, and will likely die an early, uncomfortable death.

So if you want to lose weight, eat the right kinds of foods, at the right time, and in the proper combination, and eat as much as you like, then read on. You will be pleasantly surprised at how simple it is. Lay off the high saturated fatty Franken foods, (Or as I like to refer to them FFF's), sodas, too much beer, and too many sweets, VOILA! You start to lose those unwanted pounds.

As you can probably surmise, I am not a great fan of red meat, the kind I am referring to is the commercial type that has been tampered with, in particular, beef. I do however eat a lot of fish, mostly salmon, the wild kind, not farmed. (I'll get into that later on in the book.)I am also not a fan of any highly processed food. But this does not mean you have to live life like I do. The idea here is to formulate a plan that works for you without having to give up everything you like.

If you like beef...that's OK. Just make sure it is organically raised and a lean cut and do not over cook, medium rare to rare is better. A good book to read is **"The Mad Cowboy"** written by **Howard Lyman** A cattle rancher turned vegetarian, very interesting. If you must have sweets, plan to have fewer or replace them with alternatives. I'll give you ideas later.

If you like ice cream like I do, you can always give the soy based or rice based fake ice creams a try. They taste great, they are still loaded with sugar, but considerably less fat, and you are not dealing with any dairy products which are not good for anyone except young cows. In the next chapter I will get into the fine points of a good meal plan for the rest of your life. Be prepared to be adventurous and do plenty of experimenting, you'll be surprised at just how great tasting a good diet can be.

CHAPTER THREE - "THE RIGHT NUTRIENTS"

We hear so much today about how we should

fortify our diet with nutrients from A to Z. The truth is if we ate a balanced nutrient rich diet of vegetables, fruit, nuts and grains, with some fish thrown in we would not need additional nutrients. The problem is these days our planet has been sucked dry of the nutrients essential to our health. For years soils have been depleted of essential components necessary for the production of plants that have a high concentration of vitamins and minerals.

Adding some fertilizers can help, but most create further problems and nutrients are added into our foods at the time of processing. Our food supply has been so depleted of nutrients that in order to live a normal life we now need to supplement our diet with the vitamins and minerals we should be getting from our food.

Let us examine further our relationship with food, or primarily diet, or lack of it. Diet...that ugly, ugly word we all hear far too often. Lets take a close look at what a diet really is, what makes up a diet, the affect it has on our body, and by consuming a diet suitable for us humans...the affect it would have on our planet. Diet, what really is a diet? We've heard of many, and some are just downright horrible. What does the dictionary have to say about diet?

Diet: 1. A regulated course of eating and drinking especially one followed for medical or *hygienic* . **2.** daily fare. **3.**, as regards its nutritive value or its effects on the body. To take food and drink according to a regimen. A way of living. Webster's.

Food: 1. which is eaten, drunk, or absorbed by an organism for the maintenance of life and the growth and repair of tissue. Webster's

As you can see, the sole purpose of eating is to allow the body to function properly and to be able to make repairs efficiently. If that were not the case, then why not eat just what we like to eat? As I mentioned earlier it would be lots of chocolate. How long do you think I would survive living solely on chocolate? Not too long, but I would pass with a smile on my face.

You will notice in the definition of Diet I have made bold and in *italics* the word **Hygienic**. Which means hygiene. It is probably for this reason alone that we are to consume a regular and nutritious diet. Lets take a look at the word hygiene and what the dictionary has to say.

Hygiene: 1. The science of health.

Hygiene, the science of health. Simple and to the point. A hygienic diet is a diet that is science based. For this reason we will delve into a little science, not too much as you probably aren't that interested in science as you are eating a nutritious, palatable meal. The first bit of science is quantity. How much should we consume? This is where most diets fail. They concentrate too much on calories and not enough about what kind of calories you are consuming.

Now we don't want to get into the calorie counting nightmare, but we do want to have a general idea about how many calories we consume on a daily basis. We don't want to be eating too few and become male nourished.

That would be consuming less than 1200 calories per day. (We are talking about nutrient dense calories, not sugar laden empty calories. We will touch on this later.) We certainly do not want to consume the amount of calories that say a sumo wrestler would consume on a daily basis, about 20,000 calories, most of which are fat calories.

Label reading. I understand that reading labels when you go grocery shopping is probably the last thing you want to be doing. But it is important. After a while you instinctively know what ingredients are in certain products. It is crucial to know what you are putting in your body and the bodies of your family and friends. What you eat everyday is the fuel your body needs to operate efficiently, just like your car.

You wouldn't put vinegar in the gas tank, or Gatorade instead of oil would you? Same goes for you. Once you become proficient at knowing what not to put into your body and know where to look on packaging you can streamline this process considerably. When you get to know the products you use on a regular basis, you already know what's on the label.

Back to calories. All you need to know is the average human needs between 1900 and 2500 calories per day depending on activities. Teenagers and younger ones will need more as they are growing, and growing fast. For some adults there is a program called **(Life Extension)** where adults consume only 1900 calories per day and only from good sources of raw food along with filtered water. The idea is the slight calorie restriction promotes stronger cell production making the body become younger. It is still considered a radical plan by most but makes sense once you do some research.

The average human lives approximately 75 to 80 years, women generally longer. Most humans enjoy a healthy, energetic, mobile life up to their 50's, then things can happen. For those of you reading that are not there yet (Those younger than 40sh) let me enlighten you just a little.

Without changing a moderately poor lifestyle you can expect to receive the following. Your eyesight starts to fail you. This usually happens whether or not you live a poor lifestyle or a good one. If you are living a good lifestyle it may take longer for your eyesight to diminish.

Most people start to put on extra weight, usually due to inactivity and poor diet. You may start to lose some hair, mostly men but some women too. More than likely it will also turn grey. You might have indigestion some of the time, or all the time, depending on your diet. Your muscles and bones might ache, your sleep pattern changes, you might start to forget things, usually simple things to remember. You start to make lots of excuses as to why you can't get out and do the things you used to love doing.

For some the list goes on and on. Adult onset diabetes, arthritis, osteoporosis, cancers, heart disease, Alzheimer, strokes, and obesity to name but a few. Not such a great outlook is it? So if we are to live to our 70's and beyond, (Some experts believe it possible to live to 160 years of age and in good health.) and with most of us a lot of the problems I listed previously will arise when we get into our 50's, that means we are likely to spend 20 years or more with a multitude of problems that I'm sure we would rather do without.

It doesn't have to be this way. For most of us the fix is simple, diet. It is the most important factor in living a disease free life whether you only live to 70, or live to be a hundred or beyond, you want a quality of life that you enjoyed when you were in your teens, 20's, 30's, and maybe 40's.

If we shouldn't eat big Macs, greasy pizza's, chocolate cheesecake and chips, what should we be eating? I know I'm going out on a limb here, and I'm pretty sure you know, but I'll say it again.

How about fruit, vegetables, whole grains, nuts and lean meats and fish? Sound familiar? We have all been told at some point that a balanced nutritious diet is the key to becoming and staying healthy. But over the years this balanced, nutritious diet has changed, especially in North America. We now consume far too much fat, and the wrong kind.

Not enough quality carbohydrates. Too much refined sugars. Not enough quality water. To top it off, some of us finish it all with a couple or more bad beers and a cigarette. Bad news.(More on beer, wine, and smoking later). The good news...we can change all that, and in the process start to feel better, and look better. Even the planet starts to feel better. (I'll explain later.)

Let's start with water, H2O. We humans are made up with about 75% water, everything around us is mostly made up of water. It is something we have to have everyday. And not the plain old regular stuff out of the taps anymore. (Unless you are on a well system with good water that has been tested.) This is basically lifeless water that in most places has chlorine and fluoride added. Both of these are poisons and should not be consumed in any way, shape or form.

Many cities do not test for the hundreds of other contaminants that enter our water sources. Any surface water, anywhere on this planet will have some contaminate level. Bottled water, unless in glass, is no better, and in some ways far worse. For a small bottle of water in plastic, it costs approximately two dollars to produce, about twice the price you pay. These costs are attributed to the energy required to produce the plastic, and the large amounts of water itself to manufacture the bottles. Then most of them end up in land fills, or blowing around the planet until they finally end up in the ocean and the water is generally no better than your tap water.

Here are a few things you can do to ensure your family has good water to consume and cook with. Invest in an inline multi filtering system, purchase your water in large 10 gallon food safe plastic or glass car-boys, boil your tap water, letting the heavy metals settle, and allow the chlorine and fluoride to evaporate. Then cool in the refrigerator in a large glass container and consume a glass often. Between 2 and 4, 8 oz glasses per day, depending on physical activity levels. Most of your water you should obtain from your food choices.

You say, "But John, I'll be going to the bathroom all day long." Yes, you might to start with, but that's a good thing. You will be purging your system of toxins and unwanted, left over debris that accumulates in your digestive system. Soon you won't need to go as often and your body will love it, especially your skin. Now, any questions on the water thing? Remember this is everyday.

Let's move on. Breakfast. The most important meal of the day. Why? The name will give it away...break the fast, the one you have been on for the past eight to ten hours or more. If you went that long throughout the day, you would think you were starving. A good breakfast is not a cup of coffee, or two or three, it is not a single glass of orange juice, it is definitely not bacon, some other kind of burnt meat and fried potatoes. Or, a big stack of pancakes or waffles smothered in butter then drenched with sugary syrup.

This may taste good to some people, it will fill you up, give you digestion problems, really play havoc on your entire body, and pack on the weight in unwanted fat in all the wrong places. If you are one of these people and you want to live a long and healthy life...you have to stop, NOW! I see many people who claim to be healthy and fit eat a breakfast like this almost everyday. With a meal like this you would be getting 2/3rds of your required calories per day in one meal...and a poor one at that.

Plenty of saturated fats, trans fats, and just mostly FAT! With the ever so delicious array of synthetic formulas, additives, and preservatives in most breakfast foods, if you can really call them food. Breakfast is indeed the most important meal of the day because it is the first meal upon arising from a restful sleep. What does your body want? Need? Something simple to start with, we don't want to overwork our digestive system right off the starting block.

If you have the time, breakfast should be a long and leisurely event. About an hour or so would be ideal. Leave the larger meal till mid-day with a small snack in between. This meal should not be loaded down with too many fats either. Fish is always a good protein and fat to have at any meal. A good breakfast should ideally start with fresh fruit.

Grapefruit is good, along with apple, peach, grapes, pineapple, orange, banana, dates, figs, raisins, berries, etc. Fruit should be eaten on its own before any protein. Fruit does not start to digest completely until it arrives in the lower intestines. At no time should fruit ever be eaten with sugar or any other foods. Melons, being some of the best fruit, should be eaten on their own.

In North America and other countries, we are brainwashed on how to eat our foods. We almost always have a dessert after a large meal, especially dinner. The sugars present in the fruit or other sugary treat cause problems with the digestion of other foods we consume at the same meal. Perhaps even nutritious ones. It is best to wait about thirty minutes to one hour before introducing other foods after consuming fruit. Fluids of any kind, other than a small amount of filtered water should not be taken with any meals. It is a good idea to stop drinking your fluids thirty minutes before and then resume the taking of fluids about an hour after the meal.

If you must have your morning coffee, have it thirty minutes after the fruit, wait for about twenty minutes then start drinking your water. Caffeine has a dehydrating effect on the body. If you consume more than one cup of coffee per day you should make sure you are getting enough water. When you eat fresh fruit, eat as much as you like until you feel full. Bananas will fill you up fast. You are probably wondering, where is the cereal, hot oats, whole wheat toast with preserves. I will explain later about how best to combine foods so that they are digested fully and properly.

The reason for splitting our foods into certain groups is to allow the best digestion possible. Your brain will sense the food being eaten and allow the right enzymes to be delivered to start a particular digestive process. If you find that fruit alone is just not enough, you can try a little active yogurt, that is a natural yogurt that has not been processed too much. It will also add some protein to your meal, which is important.

If you are in a hurry, put your fruit into a blender or Vita Max mixer with a little yogurt, pineapple juice, and a small wedge of lemon with the peel on. You will find yourself refreshed and feeling much better than if you ate the large greasy breakfast described earlier. Eggs can be an important part of your morning meal as long as the eggs are from free range chickens that have been fed organic, non processed feed. Not fried in butter or especially margarine.

58

If you take vitamin supplements, (Which I strongly suggest you do) make sure you take a good portion of them with breakfast to start your day out right. And make sure they are of a superb quality. We will get into supplementation later on in the book.

CHAPTER FOUR - EXERCISE

Exercise...I know, the last thing you want to hear, and you already know how important it is, on a regular basis, every day. Now the good news about exercise. In fact lets not call it exercise at all, we'll call it something like, daily activities. That's right, something you do every day anyway that you don't even think about. Walking. Yes walking, something most of us are born to do from about the age of two. Most of us have two legs that when used properly will allow us to do amazing things. Dancing comes to mind. Not only is it enjoyable to do but it also works as a great cardio workout.

But back to walking. A lot of people tell me they walk plenty when they are at home, you know...up and down the stairs, running around doing this and that. The truth is most people hardly move at all. Just have a look at most people. Far too much weight and most of it bad fat. We are living in a World where most things we do require only that we pick up a remote and push some buttons, sitting in front of the computer and TV for many hours per day.

Some people have jobs where all that is required is sitting in a chair staring at a computer screen and typing in information for eight hours a day, then back home after a two hour commute sitting in a car to arrive at home, order take out, then plunk that big ass on the sofa to watch yet another screen for four to five more hours. Who needs legs?

Have you ever seen the movie "**WALL-E**". It is a

great movie for the simple fact that it puts Humankind into the future. We have made a complete mess of our Planet and had no choice but to venture off Planet to survive on a huge spacecraft resembling a large cruise ship. All humans aboard are so fat that they are permanent fixtures in their lounge chairs.

If you seriously have a look around today it is not hard to imagine a future such as this. Let us hope not. If it were not for **Wall-e**, the small droid, Humankind would have definitely gone extinct. (That just may be my next book). We at this time in history certainly do not need the help of a little robot to get us back on track. Just get up off your fat ass and do a little walking!

But it hurts, I have bad knees, it hurts my back...well, if you start off slowly and build up to your five miles a day, those pains will likely go away and you will feel so much better you might decide to get involved with some kind of sport. We as Humans just love to make excuses, I'm no different. I constantly have to push myself to get moving more. I do not always get my five miles in everyday, I don't always do my 50 push ups, or my 20 to 30 sit ups. If you miss the odd day here or there, it will not be the end of the World. It is important however to make sure you get at least 3 - 4 days in a week.

A good book to read is **"Younger Next Year"** Chris Crowley and Dr. Henry S. Lodge, they really drill home the fact that laying around will put your body in a state of decay while lots of movement will reverse that and start to make you younger. I'm sure you have heard by now about Telomeres. They are part of your DNA and determine how long your cells will live. It was always assumed that these Telomeres were pre-programmed and that determined how long you would live. Now experts in the field are finding out that this can be reversed, and some people could actually become younger. Science is great isn't it?

Even so with all of this great science, we as humans still have to move, and move lots. Walking, OK I know you're getting tired of me talking about it, but that is how simple movement can be to start. Just find a level section, ideally a country road or trail and measure out a distance of 2 1/2 miles, pick a good time of the day for you and go for your walk...there, then back. Presto! You have done your five miles. If you are too busy, plan it with daily chores that need doing. Such as grocery shopping, picking up the mail, that sort of thing.

If you are not sure how far you have walked, I suggest purchasing a pedometer, they are cost effective and will measure your steps and give you information like how many miles or kilometres you have travelled, calories burned, time it took to walk the distance. So strap on your iPod and ear buds and enjoy your leisurely walk. With a good pair of walking shoes and loose fitting clothing, you'll start to really look forward to your daily walks.

If it is so simple you ask, why are not more people doing it? Again it comes back to that large muscle to the rear of you called the Gluteus Maximise. And I'm guessing they called it Maximise because with a lot of people it becomes very large indeed. Most of that largeness however is not muscle but fat. In some people they loose it altogether from lack of serious use. (Sitting on it for hours on end, does not count).

Walking will help with fat loss there and also strengthen the muscle. That's what it is, one of the bodies largest muscles. While you are out for your daily walk, put time aside to do a few lunges, these will further firm up the rear. On that note, stretching should always be done before your walk, and after wards. This will keep you limber for your walk, and prevent cramps and knots after your walk. Sounds simple enough, doesn't it? we're not quite finished yet. Your Heart is also an important muscle.

Without it I think we would be in a lot of trouble. So, on your walks you should take a moment to walk very briskly for about 100 feet then resume your normal gait. Do this four times for every 2 1/2 miles. This will increase your heart rate just enough to strengthen it. Kind of like doing a quick sprint to catch the rabbit. Breathing of course is important. Do your best to breath only through your nose. If you find yourself breathing too much through your mouth, slow down until your breathing is comfortable. After your fast walking spurts you will probably breath a little heavier, but once you slow back down to a normal pace you will start breathing easier.

If you find yourself walking mostly on sunny days, make sure to wear a proper sun shade hat, and avoid walking in the middle of the day. Keep your arms bare at least so you can absorb some of the suns good rays. This helps with the vitamin D absorption process, which is very good for the bones and a multitude of other functions of your body. Boy! Who knew walking could be so good for you?

If you think that running would be better for you, it can be, but I suggest short sprints worked in with your walking over long distance jogging. Long distance runners can develop a multitude of problems relating to the heavy pounding, usually on pavement and near to a source of airborne pollutants from vehicles. Many long distance runners have problems later on with their knees, and because you are constantly breathing through your mouth, your brain is getting the wrong kind of information. Not to mention the stress it puts on your heart, lungs and other internal organs that are not made for continuous exertion.

If you feel you must run all the time, or find you enjoy it, make sure you invest in quality shoes, and do your best to do your running well away from busy streets and highways. You may not realize it, but you will be breathing in massive amounts of deadly carbon monoxide from passing vehicles. This again will put stress on your system. When your heart is overworked it will put more stress on other internal functions as the heart is now commanding most of the attention and resources.

You need to protect your heart at all costs, it is one organ you cannot live without. Walking creates another benefit to your body. it will strengthen certain large bones within your body. Bones need an outside force on them to regenerate and stay strong. You won't get this benefit to your upper bones, but your legs and hips will love it.

To make sure all of your bones get the right kind of resistance it is advisable to join a gym where weight bearing exercise can be applied. Along with your walking, the least you should do at home is some push ups, pull ups, crunches, and bicep curls, along with triceps extensions using something as simple as a large can of beans, or any can of food of your choice. Just ten to fifteen minutes a day of this extra activity will keep your bones nice and strong.

For those of you that think you will have to push real heavy weights to get results, you are dead wrong. If you are experienced at weight lifting and generally lift heavy weights to meet your goals, I suggest trying this little trick, it will amaze you and you get a better muscle burn with less stress on the bones.

Take 25% of your maximum weight you generally lift and do as many reps as you can with a count of 30 seconds one way, and 30 seconds to return. With proper breathing, and taking a full minute to do every repetition, you will be lucky to get five full reps in, and your muscles will really feel like they have lifted ten times that weight.

As a previous gym rat myself, I am all to familiar with how damaging lifting heavy weights can be not only on your bones, but ligaments, and tendons as well. A little and slowly does the trick. If you feel you still want to go to a gym, that is great, just remember to take it easy, and not always listening to what others and especially some instructors have to say. Use common sense. If a part of you is hurting while doing an exercise, you should stop, or at least reduce the weight or level of intensity of the exercise.

When doing aerobics, keep it to a minimum. If you jog on the spot, have a nice soft surface to jog on and keep the time limit to about three intervals of about five minutes each. The bouncing around and movement of the arms is great, but not for extended periods of time. The place to work a sweat up is in the sauna after your exercise routine. A great way to get your walking in is a round of golf. (No Carts!) 18 holes on a nice day will get your five miles in easy. Only one caution here is that most golf courses use a lot of chemicals to get their grass to stay healthy looking and green.

I read somewhere that golfers that golf 2 to 3 times per week, and those that do maintenance on golf courses have a higher risk of breast cancer for women, and prostate cancer for men. I will cover toxins in our environment later in the book. So try and choose a golf course that uses organic systems for their maintenance.

Riding bikes can also be way to get your daily activity in. I would however recommend you ride away from roads with lots of traffic, especially highways. Just another source of chemicals your body does not need. In fact mountain biking is popular and a great workout, better air to breath, and constantly changing terrain to keep your muscles working hard, just be careful. Make sure your bicycle seat is of high quality.

Something I touched on briefly and is probably

one of the most important pieces to the puzzle is your daily water consumption. Water. One of the most single important nutrients we need on a daily basis. Second to oxygen, water becomes essential to our daily needs. How much should any one person consume on any given day? That is still up for debate.

Some experts, (Whom ever they might be) suggest that 8 to 10 8oz glasses per day. Others say about 6 to 8 glasses a day, and some are even less than that. So, who do you listen to? I personally would have to go with the fewer number than more, unless you are being very active throughout the day.

Like I said earlier in the book, I am not a scientist, Doctor, or academic. But I do understand the need to listen and pay attention to the signals your body sends out when a system in your body is required to do something. The common myth out there is if you feel thirsty, that is, your mouth becomes dry and you crave fluids. This in most cases is your first indication that you are thirsty, not dehydrated..at least not yet. When this happens, have a glass of water, and you should be alright.

Now if you are exerting yourself in hot weather for any extended period of time, your body will let you know within a short time that fluids are needed. Listen to your body, it knows. Your body is an extremely sophisticated piece of hardware. It knows what to do more than you do. That's why they are now saying that the stomach is the part of your body in charge. All too often we tend to listen to our brains, which have been bombarded with so much information, we trick ourselves into doing the exact opposite of what we should be doing.

Have you ever looked at other cultures? Even other species to see what it is they do under the same circumstances? Next time you are out playing with your dog in the back yard for hours on end on a hot summer day. Pay attention to how much water your pet laps up...not a lot. Too much water in your system can cause all kinds of problems, you can even die from consuming too much water in a short period of time.

Listen to your body, drink between 2 and 4 glasses of good water a day with plenty of water packed food,(veggies, fruit, etc.) and you will be alright. Now some good reasons to drink the right amount of water. Using less water ensures more water in our reservoirs for the future. If you drink plastic bottled water, (and you shouldn't) you will be putting fewer bottles back into the landfill systems. To keep it simple we should just do what our ancestors did, many of them lived a long and healthy life.

So now what kind of water should these four to six glasses be? Again the experts are at odds with each other. If it was about 40 years ago, almost any surface freshwater would do, but now because of heavy industry, all surface water on this planet is contaminated in one way or another. What does your city or town do? Most throw a killer cocktail of Fluoride and Chlorine into the mix, plus any chemicals from runoff from farming and industrial pollutants. Doesn't sound too appetizing does it.

There are a few places on this planet that do for the present have deep water natural systems that deliver great water without any Chlorination or Fluoridation. If you are concerned about your water source you will have to do some work at getting it clean enough to consume. On my travels to places where the water might be suspect I bring along a hand held **SteriPen** that uses light to disinfect the water. You can get more information at www.steripen.com

While still on the topic of hydration, lets talk about sports drinks. I'm sure you are well aware that the majority of sports drinks on the market are comprised mostly of sugar, water, colour then stored in a plastic bottle for who knows how long.

A good movie to watch is **"IDIOCRACY"** a movie with some frightening similarities to where our human civilization is headed, and I'm guessing in less time than the 500 years in the future that the movie suggests. Their entire economic system relied on the massive use of a product similar to that of a famous green coloured sports drink. There are other underlying messages the movie puts forth as well. I recommend watching it.

While we are on the topic of sports drinks, lets venture into the area of vitamin fortified bottled water. If you do any kind of research on how the body utilizes the nutrients that are consumed on a daily basis, you will find out that most nutrients ideally need to come from our food.(More on that later).

Vitamins and minerals need to enter our system along with food. It is not until it reaches the lower intestines that most of the absorption takes place. If it is introduced to the system to quickly, it is likely that the nutrient will pass through the system underutilized.

There are plenty of gimmicky products on the market, and as a savvy shopper you should avoid all of them. Remember, it is simple. The formula goes something like this: Consume moderate amounts of the essential nutrients, moderate amounts of quality water, enough sleep, less stress, Simple. Or so we thought. As I have mentioned earlier, navigating the seemingly endless array of fake food, medicine, vitamins, water, and exercise programs out there, it is a wonder any of us are alive. So what do we do?

I will enlighten you even more in the last chapter. For now I will try to steer you away from all of the crap our society has gotten so used to. In the next chapter I will focus on our addiction to medications and unnecessary surgeries that are so common these days. If you do the simple things, you should be able to avoid most of this unnecessary business as well.

CHAPTER FIVE - MEDICATIONS? (DRUGS)

Why we should not be taking so many man-made drugs. And when we stop taking them we....Get a better functioning system. Drugs. And that is exactly what most medications are, plain and simple. Remember when you could go downtown and see the sign...DRUGSTORE, DRUGS. In almost every town it was easy to find your drugs. The big pharmaceutical companies have been getting smarter, they now refer to them as

Pharmacy's that dispense your medications.

Let one thing be understood here, no matter how advanced we might think our science is, there is no way that human made, synthetic drugs will do our bodies any good. We are a natural species, just like all of the rest on this planet. There are now more than 70,000 different man-made chemicals on the market and counting.

When these man-made chemicals enter your body, your system first has to determine if this is something that should be in your system or not. If it is man-made, your complex biological system will not be able to assimilate it and make it work within your body. Therefore it will try to store it somewhere until it can figure out how to get it out of your system. We as humans have an amazing biological system that we continue to ignore, thinking we can outsmart nature.

Look what nature does and you will readily see that we are no match for it. We should just let nature take its course and eventually we, and many other species will be much better off.

When these drugs are stored in your body they can cause all kinds of problems and even make your symptoms worse than if you had not taken these drugs in the first place. Now your liver has to work overtime to rid your body of these toxic man-made chemicals.

So your liver is overworked and it will usually show up in the form of skin discolouration, a slight, or extreme yellowish tint. You've seen these people, they do not look very healthy, and if not addressed properly the liver will begin to shut down and express a disease all of its own.

Now don't get me wrong here, some drugs can be a life saver in an acute situation, but for long term use, most drugs will create problems within your body. Look at it like an army of soldiers always at the ready when you have been traumatized. If it is a life threatening situation your army could use some temporary help to get the problem under control. When the crisis is over, it is time for the help to leave and your bodies own army can continue on with regular maintenance and eventually heal your body.

If you are to keep adding more soldiers to the situation, your own natural soldiers will stop working as well because they are confused with all this extra help that does things a different way.

It is important to let your body do what it was designed to do, regenerate healthier cells that can fix the underlying problem.

When someone is on some kind of drug, it is common that they will be on multiple drugs. Usually one to offset the side effects of another drug. This can multiply until some people are on as many as 20 drugs or more. So what is one to do when faced with a health challenge and your doctor suggests getting on this drug, or that drug? My response would be to get additional opinions, at least three. If they are all the same, it might be advantageous to go along with the first.

Many times if the patient is living a reasonable healthy lifestyle, their own body will do the repair work and no drugs are needed. Problems usually arise when people stray from a healthy lifestyle for too long. Such as lack of proper exercise, (walking), poor diet, too much stress, bad habits, and poor sleep patterns, (Another chapter).

To make things simple, for the most part stay away from drugs. If you feel you have to take a drug, do all the research you can on how it affects the body and what kind of side affects there are, and how many. A lot of times the side affects are worse than the disease itself.

Do not be bullied into doing something just because you feel your Doctor is the educated one. Did you know most doctors are schooled less than two hours on nutrition? I personally think nutrition is a big part of how we exhibit health or illness.

A question most of us should be asking our doctors is where in there graduating class did they finish...top, middle, or bottom. You might like to know. After all, your doctor has your health, and ultimately your life in his or her hands.

As I pointed out earlier in the book, I had a very poor doctor prescribing me medications before I had been completely tested properly. After seeing a qualified doctor, I was well on my way to better health, if I had not shopped around, my very qualified doctor informed me that I most likely would not have survived more than a year. Scary stuff.

Something most of us do not do on a regular basis is read labels. Especially those labels that come with prescription drugs. As I'm sure you have seen many TV commercials about prescription drugs. They are always made to look like life could not possibly be this great without them. Then near the end of the commercial, the narrator speeds up and lists all of the side effects possible with the use of this drug. Of course at an accelerated rate of speech so no one can comprehend what it is he is saying.

Why would anyone take something to fix a problem that will more than likely create more side effects that are generally worse than the original symptom. I once was in the US and was walking through a super market looking for a few items when I picked up a bag of potato chips and read the label of ingredients, and just below that was a considerably longer list of possible side effects from consuming these chips.

I would like to say potato chips, but after reading the label I wasn't sure. The side effects could include stomach cramps, headaches, skin rash, vomiting, and the list went on...I thought how could anyone eat this stuff, let alone manufacture and sell it.

When it comes to most prescription drugs, there

are generally plenty of natural alternatives to choose from. Ones that will not create any harmful side effects and usually are considerably more cost effective. The only reason most people take these expensive and potentially harmful drugs is because their trusted doctor prescribed them and we tend to trust our doctors. After all they did receive many years of training in their chosen field.

When I was looking for a new doctor for myself, I asked many questions to make sure we were going to be a team and both do the best we could to improve and maintain my health. He openly admitted that the majority of his training was in the field of drug therapy. He was very good at prescribing drugs based on the information gathered and the symptoms expressed by the patient.

When it comes to me, we are both on the same page when it concerns the prescribing of drugs. We go in the direction of natural first. I also tend to ask a lot of questions, I have to be totally convinced and it generally involves a lot of research on the internet. It is my body, my health, and I just don't blindly put it in the hands of anyone. I think a lot of doctors have forgotten their Hippocratic oath they took, "First do no harm."

As a teenager I grew up in the 70's. The most prevalent drug around was marijuana. I had tried it and didn't like it. Now it appears that marijuana has medicinal properties, who knew? Apart from the smoke inhaled when doing it the traditional way, it appears to be a rather good way to address certain illness's.

It certainly is more cost effective if it was made legal for people to grow a certain amount for personal use only. Why are we becoming so dependent on man-made drugs? Even children as young as two years of age are now being prescribed drugs. It makes one wonder whether or not we are actually supposed to be a part of this Eco-system we call Earth.

It's amazing to me to see that out of the millions of species on this planet, only one has the need for synthetic substances to exist here. I think if we left nature to its own means we would all be better off in the long run, and a long run we may not have. For hundreds of thousands of years, we as humans have lived in balance with nature and produced strong and healthy offspring. It has been only in the past thousand years or so that we humans have managed to change a once almost perfect system to a very broken one.

Not only do we feel it necessary to drug every human on the planet, but also every other species as well. If not directly, then indirectly through our careless disposal of drugs through our water waste systems that eventually end up in the environment to cause problems with any species unfortunate enough to feed on or drink contaminated water sources.

Do you know anyone who is not on some kind of drug? Whether it be prescription or OTC (over the counter)? Not only are too many people on too many drugs, but when they have problems with the drugs they are on, the simple solution is to prescribe more drugs.

It doesn't take a rocket scientist to figure out what is going on here. Just follow the money. Drug companies, (**Big Pharma**) have so much control, and make so much money, it is not likely anytime soon that we will become a drug free society. It will really affect our children and their children in generations to come.

We do have choices though. As I pointed out earlier, if we do our due diligence and thoroughly check our health practitioners out, and ask for safer, and cheaper alternatives, we can start to bring the industry around. I am presently 55 years of age and the only pills I take are quality, clean, and scientifically formulated vitamins and minerals.

Over my lifespan to present, I may have taken half a dozen aspirin. That's it. Many people my age are on a multitude of drugs for ailments that could be cured through dietary and lifestyle changes. No cost! No side effects!

China, Japan, South America, and many more places have a very long history of curing certain ailments with plant and animal compounds. If only we here in the west could include these methods with the high tech systems being brought on the market, I think we could have the best of both worlds. This however is not likely to happen as long as the pursuit of money and power is at the forefront.

Plastic, I know it is not technically a drug, but I thought I should bring it up as it does act like a drug when the body tries to assimilate it.

Assimilate you say, yes, our bodies are bombarded with plastics daily, from off gassing to ingestion through direct food consumption, or leaching from plastic to food through heating, or the unnatural breakdown into our soft drinks, water, or processed food.

Out of all the man-made products, plastic is probably the worst of the bunch. It is a petroleum based product and has a lifespan of thousands of years. Actually, no one really knows for sure how long plastics will stay in the environment before breaking down completely.

Even when they do, what changes have they made to the balance of nature even after plastics are no more. I'm sure you have read the reports or at least heard about how plastics especially **BPA's** (Bi phenol **A**) are creating havoc with hormone activity especially in young children, boys in particular.

What is being found is that the hormone disruption is causing pre-born males to have smaller testicles with a lower sperm count. Even with boys in their early years these affects are showing up. What this will mean later down the road is far fewer males being able to create offspring. Maybe this is our way of dealing with the over population problem.

Plastic is in everything these days, our clothes, food, carpets, cars, computers, fake wood floors, building materials, toys, and the list goes on. There is however technology coming forward that can deal with some of this, so there is some light at the end of the tunnel. It's hard to believe how people could have survived on this planet sixty years or more ago without plastic. Just try and eliminate it from your life completely, not impossible, but almost.

If we continue to put foreign substances into our bodies, they have no choice but to deal with it the best way it knows how, and unfortunately that means the onset of some disease and then the crazy cycle is started.

More drugs, more problems, more drugs. Where does it stop? It stops when the majority of us question these crazy procedures and drugs and start using more natural methods to fix our health problems. Now don't get me wrong, I'm all for the new techniques for fixing acute health problems.

We have come a long way in treating burns,

fractures, open wounds, some contagious diseases, infant mortality and so on. But once these acute situations have been stabilized, we need to get on a natural maintenance program so that the body can do its magic and repair and strengthen the system.

Another form of drug that I haven't touched on yet are the dreaded cancer duo, chemotherapy and radiation therapy. With all of the information out there it is a wonder they are still being used as a mainstream treatment for cancer patients here in the west and some other countries. With a survival rate no better than those that have no treatment at all, you have to ask yourself why we even do these expensive procedures? Again, because of the money.

Cancer is a great big business and to all of a sudden find more cost effective and proven alternatives, the cancer business would practically disappear. And millions of jobs would vanish. Over the past thirty or forty years, the war on Cancer has raged. There was a time when the odd case may have presented itself, but because the lifestyle of most was healthy,

Cancer was a non issue. Really, to win the war on

Cancer all we need to do is go back to a healthy lifestyle...again, so simple. Then we could eliminate the two dreaded standard courses of treatment Chemo therapy and Radiation therapy.

If you or a loved one is faced with decisions on when and how much chemo and or radiation you should receive, I suggest looking at some alternatives elsewhere. Most clinics are outside Canada and the US for obvious reasons, if they were allowed to operate in these countries and had a better success rate than our so called traditional methods, they would soon put the big guns out of business.

It is hard for some to part with billions and billions of dollars. There are always alternatives, in many cases doing nothing other than a few lifestyle changes warrants better results. If people do not stand up and demand better health alternatives we are destined to be forced by big drug companies to submit to these barbaric procedures, it could one day become a law to go along with these treatments or face fines and jail time.

I may be getting off on a little tangent here, but all I am trying to do is get across to you the reader, that changes have to be made in order for us to survive as a species. Again, always...always, ask questions as to why, until you are completely satisfied with the answers. Do not be afraid to demand this, it is your health you are entrusting to someone else.

If you are fifty or older and are not on any prescription drugs, I applaud you. You are one of the very few these days. For those of you that are on some drug, I urge you to do some investigation and odds are you will find a better way to deal with your condition. These days with the internet we can get any information on any subject instantly and usually for free. That is also the downside.

You will invariably find a lot of information that is false. This is where education comes into play. The more you learn, the more you know and the less chance you will just go along with the status quo. It is funny how so many politicians and people of authority have waged the war on drugs for decades now.

It appears that certain drugs are OK even though the side affects will likely do you in. As long as the big drug companies are making their billions, it is

OK to have a certain percentage of patients die from the effects of the drug being used.

As I mentioned earlier my doctor had suggested the use of anti-depressants for symptoms relating to a completely different problem. Anti depressants are the drug of choice for most symptoms because it is easy to convince any patient with a complaint that they just might be depressed.

In my case, if I had gone along with the doctors diagnosis and taken the drugs prescribed to me, I am sure I would have been admitted into an asylum, and then an early death from the complications of the real problem that was causing all of my symptoms.

I understand people are busy with their lives and do not have the time to do research, get more opinions, and find extra money to cover additional costs for qualified doctors working outside of the system. Until we have a better health system with more qualified doctors who are trained in a whole body treatment process, I am afraid we will have to venture elsewhere for quality treatment for ourselves and family.

I had read somewhere that long ago, doctors were only paid while the patient was healthy. If a patient became ill, the doctor would not get paid from that patient until the doctor fixed the problem. Sounds like a good way to go, it creates an incentive for the medical field to do what it is they set out to do in the first place. Heal the body, but first do no harm.

So how does this affect our planet? With nearly half the population on drugs, and the drug companies trying desperately to get everyone on drugs, even children as young as two or three. where do you think many of these harmful drugs end up? In our rivers, lakes, and oceans.

Other species ingest them, we ingest them again as an altered man-made chemical which will cause additional symptoms, which will require more prescribed drugs to offset these new symptoms. The other species start to degenerate, and our entire eco-system is threatened. Doesn't sound so great does it?

Another alarming pattern emerging these days is the use of drugs on pets, I'm talking about antidepressant drugs and the like. Even weight loss drugs for cats and dogs! We have been consuming animals for years now that have been drugged for better production of meat, milk, and eggs.

These animals are not anywhere close to their original species, and of course we consume these drugs through the consumption of their meat, milk, and eggs. Again a large proportion of these drugs will end up in our water supply. Please...eat organic, normal cows, chickens, pigs, lambs, milk and eggs. Sure it costs more for now, but in the long run our alternative is far worse, especially for our children and grandchildren.

The best thing we can do for our children and generations to come, and our precious planet is first to admit we have done a terrible thing by letting greed and power undermine the very structure that keeps this planet and us in symbiosis. Not only admit to it, but really start to do something about it. It won't be easy, and no one will like what has to be done, but it has to be done or else.

I feel guilty, and I am guilty, along with my parents generation, their parents generation, and more than likely several generations before that. It is extremely hard not to be a part of this as with most of us it is the only way we know how to live. That would explain the blank expressions I get when talking to people about these problems.

Even now, after all of these years of trying my best to not put any drugs into my system I am at the mercy of the agricultural segment. With all of the pesticides, herbicides, insecticides being used today to grow our vegetables, wheat, corn, soybeans, and flowers, I don't stand a chance. I read somewhere that the majority of babies born in North America have up to 90% of the toxins in their bodies that they would normally accumulate in a lifetime, present in their bodies the day they are born.

We seem to have no control and it will affect generations to come. Another issue is the chlorine and fluoride that is put into our drinking water in most towns and cities across North America. Not technically drugs they are both deadly compounds on their own, and when added to the already overuse of many thousands of other chemicals, our bodies do not stand a chance. We are presently getting our wake-up call. Albeit, slowly, it is still the final warning. When will we get the big picture. Sooner than later would be better. But I have my doubts.

CHAPTER SIX - LOSING HABITS. (JUST THE BAD ONES)

Habit, Webster's Dictionary meaning;
(An automatic pattern of behaviour in reaction to a specific situation.)

I guess what we want to do here is make a pattern of behaviour that is not reactionary in a way that will have a negative impact on us and the planet. Now some habits of course are good ones, such as brushing your teeth, eating good food when you are hungry, drinking good water when you are thirsty. When the planet is in deep trouble though, we want to do different things to change a course of action.

Like not driving in your gas operated car two blocks to get some small item you could have picked up at a later date along with other things you feel you need. Not wasting water to wash your car, at least not drinking water.

There are many personal habits that can be changed to help the individual and the planet. We, as a species have become so used to throwing things away, our garbage dumps have become places for people to create full time jobs as scavengers. Not to mention other species that use our garbage as a means of food. We have become so good at being a throw away society that production of our favourite items are deliberately made inferior so that they do not last as long.

It was not long ago you could buy a TV or any other major appliance that would last 30 to 40 years! Not like today where it may last as little as five years. I often envision the day when you get all of your appliances one week, and the next week you are shopping for new ones. Great marketing.

So, watching what you purchase, and how it comes wrapped now becomes very important. The less we throw away, the better for us all, and it starts with the simple plastic bag that we are so used to using for almost everything, like grocery shopping, lining garbage pails, storing things, picking up after our pets, and the list goes on. I am sure you are now using your Eco friendly shopping bags that you use over and over and over. I have about six or seven of them and I even take one with me when I travel.

Plastic bags probably make up the majority of our throw away garbage, Apparently the **Great Pacific Garbage Patch** (a swirling mass of debris in the middle of the pacific ocean) is mostly made up of discarded plastic bags. This patch is about the size of Texas! It can go as deep as ninety feet in some places, and like I said, most of this debris is plastic, which can really cause problems for marine life when they either ingest it thinking it is some sort of food, or getting tangled up in the maze of plastic bags, plastic beer carriers, and a multitude of others.

The best habit to change would be to eliminate plastic from your life. That is a real challenge, and takes a lot of forethought. One thing you can do is when you purchase items in those plastic wrappings that are almost impossible to get off, when you do, do it in the store and leave the wrapping behind, when enough people do this, the store will have to return it to the manufacturer, who will in turn convince the packaging company to come up with a new, and Eco friendly way to package their products.

Sure, it's a little more work, but eventually we can deal with a better way of packaging. I know I mentioned this earlier, but it is probably one of the more important, and simpler things we can do to make things better.

Now to touch on some bad habits. I hope you do not indulge in these, and if you do, I would hope you would do them in a way to least affect the environment and people around you. Number one on my list is smoking. Whether it be cigarettes, cigars, pipes, or any other, if you inhale...it is bad for you. But then you already know this, it is just that this habit is probably the hardest one to quit. I had smoked for about four years when I was a teenager and was one of the lucky ones able to quit and never smoke again.

Unfortunately I have friends that aren't as lucky, and a number of them have passed on as a direct result of smoking. I can't tell you of a good way to quit, that is a personal issue, and one that will be different for everyone.

Most of the time I could care less about what one wants to do as long as they are happy and do not hurt anyone or anything else. What really bothers me is the garbage most of these people irresponsibly litter anywhere, especially on the sides of roads and highways around the world.

I recently walked a five mile distance along a rural road and counted more than 35 discarded cigarette packages. Considerably more than the discarded plastic pop bottles, beer cans, coffee cups, and plastic bags. Now think globally. To me quitting something like smoking, doing drugs, eating crap, is easy...just do it, unless you are not afraid of dying sooner than later because of it.

Alcohol, here's one I still partake in once in awhile. Which is for the most part alright for you. As long as it is in the range of no more than a couple of drinks per day, and the alcohol is of good quality without the usual suspects in it. (additives). I read somewhere that some canned beer can have as many as 90 different chemicals involved in the processing. When I make my beer it has only three ingredients. Water, hops, and malt. Wine is similar, these days a lot of it has additives to help with shelf life. One in particular.

Sulphates, can cause all kinds of problems for some people. With me, it's headaches. And no it's not because I drank too much. Quitting drinking appears to be easier to quit than smoking as a number of friends have demonstrated. They managed to quit drinking altogether, but the smoking was the hard one for them.

Smoking can have a terrifying grip on people, and believe it or not the one ingredient out of thousands in a cigarette that actually has some benefits is Nicotine, and it is precisely that one that is addictive. All of the rest of the additives are very bad for you and most do not need to be in tobacco. If you are a smoker and are finding it difficult to stop, I would suggest tracking down an organic type of tobacco, they are out there, and would be considerably better than the non organic cigarettes.

Of course the inhaling part is very hard on your lungs. Try smoking without inhaling. If we can make a conscious effort to reduce our wasteful habits we can start to make a difference to the health of our planet. Shorter trips in our cars, buy locally to reduce transportation costs, use collected water to water our gardens or wash our vehicles, combine several errands together to reduce number of trips to stores, have our children walk to and from school if within a couple of miles and the children are old enough and team up with other school buddies.

Don't leave the water running when brushing teeth, turn lights out in rooms not being used, turn down heat in rooms not being used, especially when you are away, when cooking, plan several meals in advance to reduce energy from cooking, read more books, go for walks with family and friends, purchase only environmentally safe products for you, your family, and our planet. By applying even just a few of these measures, it puts us on the right track to cleaning up our planet, and securing a better future for our children.

Habits are hard to break, but can be formed in

only about ninety days with a daily repetitive cycle. It takes some effort, but can be well worth it. So if you want the good habits, take some time to cultivate them and in the process the bad ones may just disappear.

CHAPTER SEVEN - LESS STRESS

Stress. That seemingly dirty word we hear all to often. Thing is, most of us do not understand the roll stress plays in our day to day lives. Believe it or not we all have some stress every day of our lives. Many thousands of years ago the stress most humans experienced was the Fight or Flight kind.

It was brief, and enhanced many of our priority systems in our bodies to facilitate getting away from a predator, or staying your ground to protect you and fellow tribe mates from danger. If these encounters were to last too long, the effects of the stress would eventually start to have a negative effect on some of your bodies operating systems.

Fortunately, back then these instances were few and far between and were momentary. However these days we have different kinds of stress and some of them can be perpetual. A lot of modern day stresses are small and inconsequential to us, so we ignore them and the symptoms they create.

Example: Getting into your car and taking a small trip to town and back. As soon as you get into your car, your body anticipates the stressful actions of driving on a busy roadway. This raises your heart rate, puts extra pressure on your brain functions, and creates stress hormones that can take four or more hours to subside after you return home.

Now imagine a taxi driver and how much down time he has to recuperate, virtually none. Most cab drivers work a twelve hour shift, you do the math. How about police officers, firemen, soldiers, professional athletes. I think you get the picture, is it any wonder so many of us are sick all of the time.

Most species have moments of stress, but they are short lived, then they return to a normal operating level. We humans should function in the same manner. Short, infrequent, moments of stress, such as the fight or flight stress as recognized in nature. If a stress component is ongoing it will cause underlying problems like inflammation which can lead to disease, which will ultimately lead to our early demise.

Most things we get stressed over are dealt with on a subconscious level so we are not even aware of the damage being done. For example, smoking. I know we covered that in the last chapter, but it is a perfect example of how continued stress on a system works.

Even though the act of lighting a cigarette appears to calm one down psychologically, its main stress components are hard at work destroying body parts, especially the lungs. If one tries to quit smoking this applies yet another stress upon us as we go through withdrawal symptoms. Stress has been called the number one killer in North America, and I am sure it is catching on in other countries as well.

How do we eliminate stress? We don't want to eliminate all stress, as I pointed out earlier, some stress is good for you. It can sharpen many of your senses, and actually do the heart and other organs some good. So what stresses should we try to get rid of? It should be obvious, but with our modern day lifestyles it has become one of the hardest challenges around.

We are bombarded every day with thousands of commercial messages telling us to do certain things, get certain things, save money here, spend money here, save for retirement, save for children's education, stop smoking, start smoking, eat healthy, eat unhealthy. And of course the list goes on.

The commute to work everyday for some can be as long as four hours both ways, and if all you do is sit in front of a computer all day and have to meet unrealistic deadlines, the one or two days off per week, (If you are one of the lucky ones) certainly aren't enough time to reduce your stress levels and truly relax.

Many thousands of years ago our ancestors lived a much calmer life. A few hours per day were spent on obtaining food and securing their shelter. The real only stress came from chasing down dinner, or fleeing from threats. A large part of their day

105

would involve family and friend time. They may not have lived as long, but for their time on this planet they were considerably healthier than most of us today.

Stress is a hard one to deal with when we are not even sure we are stressed or not. Generally some medical or neurological condition will present itself, and in most cases health practitioners will prescribe a drug for the symptom, not the underlying problem being stress, brought on by any number of issues.

Myself, I do my best to bring every issue into a present moment. I try not to think beyond today for most things as I do not have total control over what will transpire in the future, if I did have control over the future then I would be the King of everything wouldn't I?

You can't change the past, so don't live in it, you don't know what the future holds, so don't live in it, all you have is the moment...so live in it and make it the best you can. Eliminating stress can be an easy endeavour, if you take it one challenge at a time and don't sweat the small stuff.

If the long commute to work gets you all revved

up and stressed for the rest of the day, why not look into car pooling, or public transit, far less stressful. It may take a little longer, but you will have extra time to accomplish some daily tasks that will now free up some time on the other end. Anything that is out of your control is something you definitely need to remove from your conscious list of things to deal with.

Technology was supposed to make our lives easier, and to allow us more time to do the things we enjoy most. With cell phones, computers, up to the minute forecasting on weather and global news, advancements in medical technology. It appears now people have less time for their favourite leisure time activities.

What happened? I know many people who have worked most of their lives only to retire and find that they need to climb right back into the work force. This creates stress in a couple of ways...extra years of work for less pay for the retired person, and fewer jobs for the young as the retired ones won't cut loose.

What started out as a way to make things easier for us and give us more time to do the things we enjoy has now created a lifestyle that is far more complicated and that in turn creates more stress.

A friend of mine joked one time when I asked him if he would be retiring soon, his response was; "I'm working on having two holidays per year...six months each." We certainly need more time these days just to catch up with the fast pace us humans have become accustomed to.

Some individuals create a lot of stress out of nothing. The more stressed one becomes the easier it is to create additional stress, thus compounding the affects of everyday living. Small events like maybe breaking a shoelace are not reasons to get stressed over, some people do. In every situation remember that it has already taken place and you cannot reverse the action. We all make mistakes, some bigger than others, but once they have been made there is nothing we can do to reverse it.

It always helps me when I make a mistake to quickly step back and take a deep breath. I now realize more often than not that most things in life seem to work themselves out if given the time and patience.

Some physical stresses can be ongoing, and in that

situation it becomes difficult to completely eliminate stress. But one can make it easier for the body to cope by using the brain to produce thought patterns that can assist the body in speeding up the healing process. Our bodies are an amazing system, and if we were to allow our bodies to do what they know best, many present day health issues would disappear.

Not everyone is programmed to deal with stress in a controlled manner, some will never be able to deal with stressful situations and therefore will more than likely develop disorders of some sort. If one can learn to go with the flow and do ones best to follow the lead of nature, most everything would fall into place and make life considerably less stressful.

There are those people that resort to drugs or medications to relieve some of the symptoms of stress and anxiety, these are only temporary at best and can cause a multitude of side effects. Some forms of therapy that work are Yoga, Meditation, and deep breathing exercises. As was stated earlier, hobbies can be a very good way to relieve stress. I have several, one being writing, it always helps with a long and stressful day. Even if I have difficulty in coming up with readable paragraphs, I still enjoy the process. The brain needs stimulation, but not too much.

Multitasking might sound like a good idea, but in most cases this way of completing projects is generally incomplete and stress's the body unknowingly. Those that appear to effectively multitask usually have many tasks that are always incomplete, multitasking has been proven to be inefficient at best.

The brain is trainable and a seemingly harmless substance such as caffeine can play real games on our most complicated body part. For most people a cup or two of good quality coffee per day can be beneficial, but some, like myself do not work well with coffee or related substances. Even chocolate can have adverse effects on some.

A good goal to work towards to becoming less stressed is to reduce your heart rate. A normal functioning healthy resting heart rate should be around 70 beats per minute. Some are a little higher, and some have very low rates. A quick and simple method for determining your heart rate is to put your index finger and next finger together placed lightly on your neck just below the chin until you feel your pulse. Take a clock or your watch and time the beats for ten seconds, then multiply by 6. Now you will have your beats per minute.

You can try breathing exercises for just a few minutes then try again, you will most likely notice a drop in beats per minute. You can do this also after a session of exercise and see the difference the other way. Even doing this small exercise will improve your ability to reduce stress because you are consciously thinking about your heart rhythm and trying to lower it into acceptable ranges.

Any stress will immediately increase your heart rate, which initially in most cases is good for you. It is the prolonged stress that causes all of the health problems. It can take hours to reduce some stresses and during this time your body has to deal with it. When in a stressful situation your body slows or eliminates a number of bodily functions, such as digestion, a number of thought process's, some basic maintenance of body systems, and information retention.

Your brain is similar to your computer, information or signals are sent to it and certain responses are then performed to many of your bodies operating systems. You can think of your brain as the foreman of the operation and delegates work to the workers, your cells. You might think that your brain is the all important organ of your body, but it really only does what it is told to.

When you are stressed your body sends the signals to your brain to start the flight or fight response that is built into virtually every species on this planet. When that happens for prolonged periods of time, your brain will not send out the right commands to optimize your repair and regeneration systems. When this happens, chronic inflammation sets in and over time can result in disease.

Any stress on your body should only be for limited time frames so that regular maintenance can be performed as necessary. If there is continual inflammation in some region of the body, symptoms arise and eventually disease, and unless the underlying problem is relieved the process continues and of course the disease worsens and spreads to other internal or external systems.

This is often the case with cancers. Stress will take its toll if not kept under control. Physical stress's are also an issue when it comes to overall health. Let us take a marathon runner as an example. Most people would think that this type of athlete would be in excellent shape and have very few health issues. Only if the running athlete is on an extensive nutritional program to assist in rejuvenation.

Unfortunately the constant stress on heart, lungs, muscles, ligaments, and tendons will ultimately take its toll. Our bodies were not designed for extended intervals of excessive physical activity. We need time to recuperate. Down time for our system to regenerate for the next flight or fight. An example would be other species and how they deal with everyday stress's.

Watch a dog, or a cat throughout its day and you will notice that they spend a lot of time resting. This gives them the energy and power required to chase down their dinner. Most species do not have the unique capabilities of us humans. We are somehow able to take a very simple situation and create an endless succession of more involved problems stemming from this seemingly minuscule challenge.

We humans seem to thrive on creating a challenge

113

out of thin air. Most times this will cause undue stress on not just one person, but many who are close to the perceived problem. It takes time and a lot of work to change the habits that have been instilled in us from an early age. It is however important that we take the steps necessary to overcome these trained habits.

It is said that it takes about 90 days to form a new habit, so to replace a bad habit with a good one will take about that same time frame. repetition is the key. Just like brushing your teeth, something we do everyday. The closer you can get to living in the now, the easier it is to deal with situations that arise in the future. Nothing is so bad that it cannot become a stepping stone to a more stress free future.

Some people have told me that in order to live a life with little or no stress, one must have faith. I guess that is true, I am not a religious person in a traditional sense, but I do have faith in the eventual enlightenment of humankind in the grand scheme of things.

Our limited knowledge of how expansive and complicated this universe is leads me to believe that there is only one way for the future to go, and that is in a positive direction. It is only logical. So with that in mind, it only makes sense for one to yield to forces beyond our control and enjoy the moment for what it is.

Another form of stress which is now becoming common place is something called dirty electricity or **EMF. (Electric Magnetic Field)**. We are surrounded by millions of these fields coming from simple everyday appliances such as microwave ovens, microwave towers, cell phones, cordless phones, computers, TV's, X-rays, Power lines, and certainly many more. So how do we deal with this form of stress? It becomes very difficult if you are dependent on your phone and or computer for your profession.

The best place to start eliminating these forms of dirty **EMF's** in your bedroom. We have become so accustomed to having such things as cordless phones, computers, radio alarm clocks, TV's, fans, electric blankets, stereos, and other forms of electrical items. Your bedroom should be a place for sleep only. It has only been in last forty to fifty years that some of these electronic devices have made their way into our one quiet place where your body and mind can recover from the days destructive forces such as stress, anxiety, and an assortment of toxic substances taking their toll on our bodies.

Sleep is probably the most important part of our daily routine. Something I will get into later on in the book. Keeping your home **EMF** free can be a challenge, but the bedroom can be a place of solitude and only to be used for sleeping. The rest of the home becomes more difficult.

A media room is ideal for all electronics involving listening to music, watching TV, being on the computer, and playing video games. Keeping a minimum number of cordless phones in the home can help, and have at least one phone directly wired so as to keep **EMF's** getting too close. In the kitchen I would suggest eliminating the micro-wave altogether and relying more on convection ovens for quick
heating.

There are meters you can get to measure the dirty electricity in your home, or you can get a qualified technician in to do a thorough system check for you.

Many of us tend to jump from one **EMF** zone right into another, our vehicles. We have the stereo, cell phone, and sometimes a laptop all within a close proximity to us as we drive to and from work, or on other excursions away from home. Some vehicles even have several monitors for viewing movies or the internet. A lot of people are never away from these forms of **EMF's.**

Any electrical field that is close enough will interrupt our normal electrical field. As we know, our electrical field is very important to the proper functioning of every system within our body. If it wasn't for a proper functioning electrical system, our hearts would stop, and our brains would short out. In fact there have been reported cases where certain individuals have had small electrical explosions within their brains. Sound like the twilight zone? Who knows for sure.

An important daily ritual to help with all of this negative energy infiltrating our complex system is to wind down and take about twenty minutes each day to completely relax and allow our bodies to release and reboot, just like our computers when they get too bogged down with far too much irrelevant information. Down time is so important to our overall health. Not only mental, but our physical.

If stress is permitted to reside in our bodies it will continually degrade our intricate system by attacking week spots that most of us have. This can advance many chronic disease's that will ultimately take its toll and sometimes result in death if not intervened in time. Chronic inflammation can appear anywhere in our bodies. Resulting in many different symptoms from aches and pains, to rashes, and digestive problems.

Most doctors will prescribe drugs to alleviate the symptoms and not address the underlying cause's. With more than 70,000 man made chemicals in our environment it is only logical to assume that many of them will get into our food, air, and water sources. When physical and mental stress's invade our bodies the damage is almost immediate. It will then progress to the point where it shows as a symptom of something more serious that if not dealt with properly will manifest into something considerably more problematic.

As expressed earlier in this chapter, reducing stress at every point is the key to better health. By reducing the stress on ourselves, will reduce the stress to our planet. Habits such as smoking, consuming too much alcohol, and drug dependency are all forms of acute stress that should be avoided at all costs.

I know it is difficult for many to stop some of these habits, I used to smoke, drink too much, and do drugs. I was fortunate that I could quite, and reduce these habits so my body had a chance to regenerate at a healthier level. I would have to say that smoking is without a doubt the most difficult habit to quite. I have lost many friends to this killer habit.

The strange part is that by justifying the act of lighting up a cigarette, having another drink, or just one more hit, seems to relieve stress momentarily, but we know that the underlying damage will create much more stress than the body is capable of dealing with in the long haul. One day at a time, and one small step in the right direction can do wonders for ones health. Especially for ones mental health. Just start with one positive action per week and keep doing it for no less than ninety days so that the habit becomes automatic. Within a year, you are well on your way to creating a better you and better planet for us all.

CHAPTER EIGHT - SLEEP

AND REST

Ahhh...a good nights sleep, we all need it but how many of us really get it, and what constitutes a goods night sleep? Most of us have been told that eight hours should be the ideal amount of time. Some of us do well will fewer hours, and others seem to need more than eight hours. Myself, I seem to do best with about nine hours of sleep per night.

Of course the nine hours are not entirely made up of the deep REM sleep needed to allow us to wake up refreshed and full of energy. Everyone is different and to get the best of your time when trying to sleep not all environments need be the same. Studies suggest that those who get fewer than seven hours of sleep per night have a tendency to put on and keep more weight than those that get more hours of sleep.

Part of this might be due to the fact that with more hours of sleep one has less time to eat more food.

Those that tend to retire late, any time after ten PM also tend to eat snacks late into the night and with less time for your body to deal with this extra calorie load, it becomes difficult to burn calories and keep your weight down.

With less sleep your brain does not have time to slow down and deal with only those functions that are automatic. With too much information streaming in and out of your thought process, getting quality and beneficial sleep is practically impossible. With more stress, there is an inconsistent rhythm that your brain has to deal with.

Slowing down before getting your nights sleep is crucial to allowing your brain to wind down after a busy day. One of the problems people have that get fewer than seven hours sleep per night is they tend to have a non schedule for eating meals. This means they tend to snack at odd times especially late at night which is probably one of the worst times to eat. They don't call it break-fast for nothing.

The time you are at rest allows your body time to deal with all of the days physical and mental stress's. To all of a sudden introduce another round of calories to the mix can cause all sorts of problems, one being a weight problem. It is a good idea to abstain from eating any foods after eight o'clock in the evening.

A regular eating schedule is important and restricting calories later in the evening send signals to your body that sleep is soon to happen and the maintenance crew can prepare for the night shift and do all of the repairs necessary. If you must have a snack before going to bed, make it something easy to digest, and keep it small. I find sometimes I feel hungry in the evening, but a glass of filtered water seems to curb the hunger and I can get a good nights sleep.

Where you sleep and what you sleep on is a crucial component to the sleep equation. I prefer a firm mattress, where others prefer a softer one. I also find now that I am getting older I sleep better if I have a slight incline so my head is slightly higher than my feet. I was told once by a mattress salesman that our ancestors used to sleep in a sitting position. Reason being they could get to a standing position quickly if they were being threatened.

Placement of your bed in your room is also

important. Certain Asian countries believe placement of not only the bed, but everything else in your home is important to a calm and peaceful living space. Ideally you want your head to be close to a source of fresh air as many homes these days have many construction materials that are releasing toxic compounds.

Anything with a plastic smell to it should be removed if possible. Another is removing anything electrical such as radio's, cordless phones, TV's, electronic alarm clocks, electric blankets, and any computer equipment. We went through this earlier with the EMF's. For some I will suggest that a room humidifier or DE-humidifier can be helpful if you experience dry eye, dry throat, or you snore frequently even people that are afflicted with POCD can benefit from a steam vaporizer.

Your bedroom should only be used for the purpose of sleep. It should be as dark as you can possibly get it, and as quiet as you can possibly get it. Your body has a natural sleep and wake cycle that is tuned into the natural day and night rhythm of nature. People in Northern climes have during the summer months almost no darkness, which makes for some sleep deprivation issues.

On the other end they also have very long winters where daylight is very scarce. The use of light therapy is popular to ward off bouts of depression that can lead to chronic problems for many. Those in Southern climates have a better dark to light ratio, generally about 6 AM - 7 PM.

That is probably why so many feel better in southern climes. Napping, for those of you that like to take naps, it can be a good thing as long as you keep the duration of the nap to no more than twenty minutes. Any longer and your body will think it requires more sleep and will start the process you should be experiencing when you retire for the night.

Attaining REM sleep. (Rapid Eye Movement) The part of sleep that is most beneficial. Naps can be a great quick fix for a small deficiency in quality sleep that was interrupted the night before. Early to mid afternoon is a good time to lay down for a rest if you feel the urge. You don't even need a dark and quiet room, it is how ever preferable.

You will not get into REM sleep, but your body

will have enough rest to give you a bit of a burst of energy to carry you through the rest of the day. Even a short rest while commuting on a train or bus can help. Just remember to keep it short or you may go through the rest of the day feeling sluggish.

Most other species seem to have a real knack for napping, again just watch cats and dogs, they are very good at getting a little shut eye throughout the day. Of course with a good seven to nine hours of productive sleep per night a person should be able to navigate through the day just fine without any down time.

I have had many jobs in my life that required a great expense of energy throughout the day, and most of them were outdoors so there was plenty of fresh air to keep me energized. For those of you that get into a car early in the morning and commute to work for an hour or more, spend your day seated at a desk for about eight hours, then return home in rush hour for the ride home. This sets you're body up for many health issues.

Your body was designed for movement, and to get plenty of movement throughout the day requires a schedule where movement becomes necessary and because of this your body will want adequate rest so it can regenerate for the following day. If you have no option when it comes to your work schedule, find ways to incorporate movement into your daily routine. Even simple movements at your desk can help. Ideally a ten to twenty minute walk would be best.

Another robber of quality sleep and rest is Sleep Apnoea. Even just regular snoring throughout the night can cause many health issues with individuals and their partners, who can many times lose sleep because of the incessant noise throughout the night. The main culprit to snoring is additional fat. Lose the weight and many times lose the snoring. Often your bed may be the culprit. Sometimes elevating your upper body slightly can help alleviate breathing problems.

It has been suggested that a cool mist humidifier can help a host of sleeping issues. This is a low cost solution and non toxic of course. Many people who snore, have asthma, or COPD, have claimed to have positive results with this low impact solution. Just check out your appliance dealer to find the one best suited for you.

People who use sleeping aids such as sleeping pills, (Those of the man made chemical type) will experience sleep, but not a restful sleep. Your body is a highly advanced biologic system that knows what to do, and when. Many times when people have problems sleeping it could very well be environmental, even something as simple as to whether or not it is a full moon, or new moon.

Many times on just such occasions I have difficulty in getting sound sleep, or the opposite where I get a very good nights sleep. I always let my body do what it wants. I do not let my brain get in the way of things. The most I would ever do is take a safe, and organic type of Melatonin, and then it is only when I have disrupted my sleep pattern as when flying across many time zones. Or, as I have recently just done, spend a week or more on Buses and Trains as I travel around the World.

Other stand buys might be a warm glass of whole organic milk. As much as I disagree with its consumption. My Mother always suggested something sweet before you retire. Not sure if it ever worked or not, but it always tasted good. There are probably as many different solutions to getting some sleep as there are people who sleep. If you have your own ritual that doesn't involve drugs or large amounts of fatty food, why change anything. In the long run it is more important to get a good nights sleep than worry about a few extra calories.

While we are on the topic of calories, a great way to get your body and brain ready for some good sleep is to do some light exercise about an hour before retiring. I like to do my push ups and sit ups before I go to bed, then read a few chapters of a good book. As I mentioned earlier, your place for sleeping should be just that, for sleeping only. All other activities should be done in separate areas of your home.

The TV is probably the worst culprit. These days people have TV's in almost every room...even the bathroom, which is fine, as long as it is not in your bedroom. I have been guilty of this practice myself. What a TV does to your brain in the subconscious can alter many brain patterns, sleep being one of them.

The exception to this rule would be a good book, one that does not involve too much grey matter to decipher. That would explain why children do so well with getting to sleep when they are being read to. Sit them in front of a TV, and they get wound right up.

A steady audio frequency can also produce the right environment for restful sleep. I am sure you have heard of the many audio programs you can get like a rolling surf, waterfall, wind through trees. A lot of these audio programs work well for meditation as well. Of course the only drawback is the electrical component which can cause negative currants within the sleeping area. The best is a completely quiet and dark room. This can be a challenge. As most rooms in any home have multiple devices that require electricity.

A new terminology with electricity in the home is called dirty electricity which can cause all kinds of health problems. There are devices that can be purchased to reduce these harmful electromagnetic fields and you can also have a person come into your home and check to see how much dirty electricity there might be in your home. Remember, simple is always best when it comes to any household appliance or convenience.

I would suggest a completely separate room for meditation and winding down for the day, so that

130

when you are ready to retire for the night your body will be ready and sleep will come quickly. Most people work early in the day and therefore think they need an alarm clock to wake themselves. I found this not to be true. I had used an alarm clock most of my adult life up until the age of about forty.

I had been working as a cab driver in Whistler BC Canada and was working the day shift which started at between 4 - 4:30 AM sometimes six days per week. I have never been a really early morning person and detested alarm clocks as they always startled me into a half waking kind of stupor. I did not function well for at least three to four hours after, and the fact that I was driving a vehicle for 12 hours or more put my body into a lot of undo stress.

I decided to train myself to work without an alarm clock. I had read somewhere that internal suggestions, repeated a few times before turning the lights out to go to sleep could instruct the brain to wake at whatever time you repeat to yourself. I gave it a try.

The first morning I awoke about ten minutes

before the suggested time the night before. I was amazed, was it just luck or coincidence? To this day from that point, I have never set an alarm clock to wake myself, no matter what time it might be. Give it a try. The simple act of ageing can play havoc on ones sleep. When we are young, sleep just seems to come naturally, and so it should as we get older.

What we fail to understand is that children tend to sleep better because they have fewer outside influences to distract and compromise their natural body chemistry. What us adults do is to take on far too much in the way of outside stimuli that keeps our brain engaged for far too long.

As I write this section of the book I am in Portugal, a rural area just outside of Portameo on the southern coast. I am presently working on an organic farm that provides room and board for some work done on the farm. It is called **WWOOFing**, a worldwide organization to put small farmers in contact with cost effective help.

I have found that the laid back attitude, and non stressful lifestyle along with a very good vegetarian diet promotes an environment perfectly suited for proper sleep. There are literally no sounds of any sort throughout the night, even the rooster next door waits until noon before he crows.

For a big part of my adult life I have had the constant noise of highway traffic, I don't think I ever got used to it and always figured I was a light sleeper. Now experiencing a truly full nights sleep I feel better rested than I have for years.

So many adults use prescription drugs to handle their sleep deficiencies and then wonder why they do not feel well. You would not think of giving your child a sleeping pill if they could not sleep. You would just read them a story, or if it was early, to play with them to tire them out. Maybe we should follow suit.

Many people have the ritual of TV, I will not suggest you remove this entirely from your life as there are many programs that are beneficial. I would just caution you to keep it to any other room than your bedroom. My Grandparents did not own a TV until the 80's. Before that, card games, putting puzzles together, listening to music, and reading were what worked well for a good nights sleep.

If you are a self employed person often work will follow you home or maybe you work entirely out of your home. This takes extreme self discipline to schedule work related projects with a well balanced home life. Put children into the mix and you have a whole new ballgame. A good strategy for getting the body and brain ready for a good nights sleep is to take a twenty to forty minute light walk after your last meal. Keep it light though, we just want to get a little fresh air and some movement to help with digestion.

Something of concern for some is the constant feeling of exhaustion, even after having sufficient hours of sleep per night. If this continues for any length of time it would be a good idea to contact your health practitioner. Some of the culprits could be drugs that have been subscribed to you, even the sleeping pills you might be taking to get yourself to sleep.

Lack of beneficial sleep could also be linked to diet and possibly food allergies. Again, people who eat late at night generally eat a poor choice of foods. Dairy for most people can cause upsets through the night, coffee is another. I suggest staying away from a heavy consumption of meats before retiring.

As I am writing this chapter I am still in Portugal and it took me about a week to adjust to the time difference, about 8 hours different from Vancouver. If you travel a lot and through many time zones it is best to set aside a suitable amount of time to adjust, and during this time keep meals light with enough good water.

Since you are travelling to other places, your sleeping accommodations will vary from that which you are accustomed to. Mattress's of different hardness, pillows being different, temperatures not being the same, lighting, noises such as traffic, dogs barking, sirens, the close proximity of people talking late into the night. All of this can take its toll.

Just remember to take it easy and not get to stressed about the occasional missed few hours of sleep. More than likely in most cases it can be attributed to the days events beforehand. If you feel your present job may be interfering with your regular sleep pattern, and it will be long term, it might be wise to re-evaluate your chosen profession. Life is too short to get caught up in something that will shorten your life and more than likely make you sick.

It was only a few thousand years ago that humankind actually had it figured out. Work about three to four hours per day to obtain your food and maintain a suitable lodging. The rest of the day could be spent socializing, the pursuit of artistic endeavours, and hobbies. Who ever thought of the eight hour a day, five or six days per week work routine must have been out to lunch. Remember..."The only true wealth in life is your Health." Go ahead, sleep on it for a while.

CHAPTER NINE - POSITIVE ATTITUDE

Attitude. **"A** *complex mental state involving beliefs and feelings and values and dispositions to act in certain ways. "He had the attitude that work was fun".* **(Webster's Dictionary).**

We all have one, some have a better one than others, and because everyone is different, no one attitude is alike which makes for some challenging situations in life. Someone might say that that person has a negative attitude, but just maybe it is a more realistic one than that of the person judging. If one is constantly dwelling on the negative and very seldom sees any positive, especially if one negates the auto responsive reaction of laughter, then yes, this could be an issue that puts unnecessary stress on many bodily functions.

People that are chronically negative day after day, year after year tend to live shorter and obviously unhappy lives. Then on the other end of the spectrum is the Pollyanna effect where a person thinks that everything is rosy and will always work out regardless of the circumstances.

This is living in a non reality type life. Sure, It would be great if everything was perfect in our World, but it is not, and I believe the reason is we need some challenges to come our way periodically so we know the difference between the two and can make an intelligent assertion based on the relative information at hand.

It is unfortunate that there is crime, hunger, abuse, and unfair circumstances. But if there weren't, how could we possibly make an educated evaluation of the matter at hand. We need opposites to make the good work. So as healthy as it may seem to have a positive outlook on everything, and disregarding the negative, that way of thinking will come back to haunt us in many ways. I am not sure how everything works in this weird and wonderful place, and when you bring **Quantum Physics** into the equation one can get very confused.

But I do feel that overall, good has to be the direction we take as a species, it makes sense and ultimately leaves the longest lasting feeling. The important thing to remember is to keep our ego's in check and know that we are a small piece of a much larger puzzle.

When it comes to health, and especially weight control, attitude definitely takes front row. You can do almost anything right, but if you are not thinking right, all is for nought. Many times someone will ask me about how certain actions may play out when applied. I say, "I don't know, we'll see." The reason for this is an attitude of submission to the powers that be, the powers we cannot change, and should not even try to.

When it comes to competitive sports, attitude plays a very large roll. Some would say that competition is counter productive. Possibly, but given the right attitude it can be very exhilarating and beneficial, if again executed with the right kind of attitude. I have played competitive sports, and it is extremely difficult to suppress certain negative thought patterns from infiltrating an otherwise positive thought process.

Especially team sports, where there are so many different attitudes. This is where the coach comes in, if the coach has a balanced attitude and is not so concerned about the outcome of the game, he or she can concentrate on how to bring the team together in a unified thought process, attaining the same attitude towards the game at hand.

If a team can achieve superior results through a combined practical and positive attitude, just think what one can do individually, especially with ones health. I have adopted an attitude of, 'things turn out the way they do for a reason,' and that reason is beyond my present understanding of how things work in this universe. I cannot change the past, and I have no certainty of the future...all there is, is this moment. So to keep from blowing a gasket over what might appear to be monumental circumstance to overcome.

I again believe they are happening for a reason, and that reason is a positive one to allow me to move in the right direction to solving the mystery of even life itself. Sound a bit too heavy? I tend to agree, that is why I leave it for the most part in the back of my mind and enjoy the journey.

Many people when faced with options, decisions, even information from a second hand source, will arrive at an unsubstantiated conclusion that usually involves a negative perspective. Example; *"Aunt Harriett called this morning."* Many people would often say something like; "Oh, *is she alright?"* Or the news station is talking about the weather in another part of the Country; "Oh my

Gosh, that's terrible!"

We have to understand that there is no terrible, or alright, it just is. Of course this gets back to **Quantum Physics** , a very involved set of parameters even the highly educated Physicists do not understand. Programming the brain with a constant flow of negative possibilities will undoubtedly result in a short circuit somewhere, and the time spent here virtually completely wasted.

As I said earlier, I believe we are here to learn and grow, or become more enlightened, from here we will continue in some aspect as a more positive flow of energy, which is all we and everything else really are.

OK, enough of the heavy stuff, how does this help with my health, and that of the planet? Knowing that everything in this World is in flux and never for a moment staying constant helps to ground one in believing that nothing is forever and that to take things too seriously can affect our health, and because of those defensive actions the planet will also suffer through our actions. Remember the saying; *"Don't sweat the small stuff, it's all small stuff."*

141

Even in the larger scheme of things, because everything is changing it means that somewhere down the road the issues that had got you all stressed out have now changed and have no bearing on how you handled them in the first place.

My Grandmother often said to me after I had asked the question; "*What do you think of all of this new technology and the way the World is headed?*" She would say; "*Everything changes...all the time...at the same time, which is now.*"
She was a smart woman, I never saw her stressed out. She had a great attitude.

A good attitude is something young children have. Sure they have their moments, but shortly thereafter they are laughing and having a good time because the future has no meaning to them, only to older children and adults because it is instilled in us that there will be a future and somehow we are supposed to do something now to affect it down the road.

When I was a young boy of about 6 or 7, I very

much wanted to be an astronaut, I still do. Then I wanted to be a cowboy, still do. A rock star, a movie star, and author, and the list goes on to this day. I want it all. Some say I should have settled into a regular job and put away for my future.

How was I to do that if I did not know what the future held for me. As I write I am 55 years young and in great shape, no medications or drugs of any kind. I feel if I had gone the usual route of many, my health would have suffered.

To many this lifestyle would be stressful and possibly have a negative effect on their stress levels. That is the key, keep stress levels low no matter what. I was up in a small plane not too long ago and it was the first time in a small plane in about 25 years.

The pilot kept asking me if I was alright, and how was my stomach. I responded..."*Fine, I feel fine.*" And I did, I am sure my pulse rate never got above 70. I felt very calm and at ease. Now you say sure what if the plane were to go down and possibly crash? Well, I am sure I would get stressed to some degree which is a good thing.

Stress can focus the senses and help in many

situations where a clear and sharp mind are important. A good attitude towards acute and critical situations. What I am trying to get across here is that a reasonable attitude to every situation that surfaces will help with dealing with the perceived problem. The right kind of stress can help, and the wrong kind can cause all kinds of problems, especially with ones health which may not surface for years after.

I've always been amazed with people that can keep calm and collected in any situation, they are few and far between and it makes you wonder what it is they do to remain that way when faced with so many difficult decisions.

Again I am sure it comes down to attitude and dealing with only the closest and immediate challenge at hand, not being concerned with the entire situation and all of its components. That is why trained Fire and Rescue, Police, Soldiers, and personnel in careers like that are calm and focused on the matter at hand.

Of course this can take many years to perfect and generally in completely foreign situations this person may become confused and unstable. What can be learned from this? It takes daily training in all kinds of situations to become comfortable and think straight.

Being able to look at something and run the process through until one has enough information to follow through on a plan of action to facilitate a beneficial outcome. No one said it would be easy.

If we are to be in this place for approximately eighty years or so, why not take the time to try and understand more of what transpires around us on a daily basis. I read somewhere that most people sit in front of a TV for more than two months of the year, add onto that the time behind the wheel going to and from work about 25 more days and one can certainly see there is plenty of time to incorporate positive habits into ones lifestyle.

As I look out to the ocean view I have here in Albufeira, Portugal from the apartment I am staying in, there is no TV, but the view certainly makes up for it, and it allows me to get plenty of writing done. Looking out over the ocean always makes me feel good inside, and my commuting now is done entirely with my own two legs...oh, that's what they are for.

Since I have been travelling certain things have improved for me. I have lost weight and have not been in great shape like this in years, and my mind seems considerably clearer. Not knowing what to expect at any given moment, and having no concrete travel plans has put me in a position of low stress. I do not have to think about where or what I should be doing or going at a particular time. It reduces any bad stress by large amounts. I can truly enjoy what the local surroundings have to offer.

Many people have a hard time being spontaneous, I find it exhilarating. Of course it is easier to do when you travel alone, as I am doing on this adventure. Developing a carefree attitude can be very liberating, it gives you a real sense of freedom, but you have to accept things mostly as they are, you cannot go about trying to change everything to suit your needs. If you do, it will backfire and put undo stress on you and your body and negate any positive advances produced. I have met a few people doing exactly the same thing, mostly women. They have put everything in their lives on hold, or have adopted an entirely new life, in a different place.

Many people I meet ask me how I can live this

way, my response is, how can I not. We Humans now for a very long time have tried our hardest to change everything surrounding us, it does not work. We could be so further ahead in every way if we were to acknowledge the power of nature and to work with it.

If we were to adopt an ancient way of living like those of the Hunter Gather's along with a modest attempt at farming, and work within the rules and regulations set forth by nature we could have so much more than we do now, and the planet would be so much better off, and of course with that we would also be better off psychologically and health wise.

Unfortunately we have an ego problem that just won't go away and we are hell bent on trying to fix something that is not broken. This would account for all of our bad stress and mostly poor attitudes. When I was being brought up as a child I was being taught how to get along with others, as I have four siblings. We were taught to respect others and other living things, to conserve, to live a simple but productive life. Offer something of value to the community.

I am not suggesting we limit ourselves. I am a

strong believer in technology and feel if we can manage our resources better and take care of our planet, the future could be very wonderful indeed.

To accomplish a symbiotic relationship with our home planet we need to incorporate biological components to our technology and discontinue the rapid depletion of valuable resources such as water, forest, and other species. We need to adopt the attitude of caregiver first, not taker of everything at any cost. This unhealthy system we have put in place will ultimately end in chaos and destruction.

The signs are right in front of us, yet we continue to ignore them. Your attitude is everything. It determines your everyday choices that ultimately will affect you and your health and that of the planet. So why not start making small changes today, it does not have to be much, maybe when shopping make the decision to not use plastic bags, instead bring a bag of your own that is made from a non destructive product.

This small action starts something within that will overflow into other aspects of your life and you will find yourself automatically doing more to help clean up this mess we have all put ourselves into.

Our two main goals should be to wean ourselves off of fossil fuels, and to reduce the Human population of this Planet. I read in one of my many books on the topic of over population that an ideal number of Humans living on this planet would be between 500 million and one billion tops. With a population base with these numbers every Eco system would be far healthier, including ourselves.

So why is it we continue to over populate and create so many dysfunctional systems that destroy the very thing that will help keep us healthy and surviving over millennium? Money. The creation of it, the collecting of it, the hording of it.

The accumulation of money serves no purpose other than to feed a few over inflated egos. Those with attitudes that are of a complete opposite configuration needed to keep this planet healthy and functional. Take money out of the equation, and everything will normalize. The Planet will come back to a point of homoeostasis and all species including ourselves will become healthier.

149

Over many of thousands of years, ours, and many other species because of our meddling have become inferior. Our basic make up has been compromised and with every succeeding generation we become more fragile.

Sure, our life span seems to have increased, but as a famous genetic biologist Dr. Myron Wentz says; "We are living too short, and dying too long." Meaning many of us are drugged to a point where we only exist, there is no life to speak of. Life needs to be lived fully, doing something of benefit to one and the surrounding environment. If not, this person is only taking up space. I know that sounds over simplified, but this is the way nature works and has worked for millennium.

Our attitudes towards such things as life and death will have to change if we are to survive and thrive in generations to follow. We callously throw lives away while doing our utmost to save lives that should not be saved.

Nearly 30,000 children die everyday from illness's related to malnutrition. This only seems to bother but a few people. I won't even get started on other species. Not anyone said that living on this planet was going to be a cake walk. It has its challenges and always will. It is necessary for life to truly evolve, it is not an overnight plan, and I firmly believe that we are not to be messing with something as Involved as nature is. It seems simple enough, pick up after ourselves, keep a tidy living space, don't pollute our water, food, or the air we breath. Kind of like the Hippocratic oath Doctors make; "First do no harm." The reason I continue on this track is to express my concern not only for our home but for the overall health of every other species, mostly our own as we appear to have the ability to be creative and make decisions that can alter many crucial components of this amazing thing we call life.

By doing simple things to bring things back to what they once were we will start to eliminate the harmful stress's that can and do affect us all. We have to, or all is for not. I pay close attention to detail when it comes to health. I have been allowed to use this body of mine, and I am thankful that I was given a reasonably good one.

There was no contract that I am aware of, but from an early age I could only assume that I was to take care of it, and take care of it the best I could. Don't get me wrong, there were definitely times when I had abused and mistreated my body, but for the most part I have taken reasonably good care of it.

I am 55 years of age at this writing and am on no drugs of any kind including what they consider safe drugs. (Medications). There are a few that can save a life in an acute situation, but long term on any kind of drug or harmful substance will cause undo stress on the body and mind.

If we want a healthy Planet for our children to grow up on then we must all make some fundamental changes to our lifestyles. The argument here is that everyone works hard during their life so that they can have the good life when retired. Look around, how good is the good life if you have to lie to yourself about the state of our home, this Planet.

A saying from Earl Nightingale I rather much like and holds a certain truth to it; "Most people tip toe through life expecting to arrive at death safely." Life is to be lived full throttle. I know a few who have lived a safe life and are now so afraid of dying they continue to do everything in their power to stay alive.

I thought the whole idea of living would bring

you to death with multitudes of experiences to share to younger generations so that they might learn. I am afraid all our younger generations are going to learn is how to mix your meds just right so you can avoid death at all cost.

I know it sounds a bit bleak, but it is today's reality. And it does not paint a very optimistic picture of the future. There are small pockets of people who are indeed doing things right, but it will take the efforts of all of us humans to get the train turned right side up and back on the track heading in the right direction. Simple things like adopting the attitude of doing your best not to use plastic, turn off lights when leaving a room, better yet, install motion sensors.

Understanding that the energy efficient bulbs we are told to use instead of incandescent bulbs ultimately will hurt our Planet and of course we humans because of the Mercury used in the production of fluorescent bulbs. Combining errands to minimize trips in vehicles, walking more instead of driving, eating better produced foods, the list can go on for a very long way. It takes people taking responsibility and doing the research to help understand how our complex economy works. It is not all death and destruction...but it could very well be if we make no changes.

I have a hard time with trying my best and then right alongside of me someone has thrown garbage out on the street, or flicked a cigarette butt out the window of a gas guzzling vehicle. Why do we do it? The formula can be so simple and then everything starts to respond in a good way. Life becomes better for everyone and everything. Some people believe it is a test, some believe it is just the way it is supposed to be, and others believe we need the challenges to grow and make ourselves better. I wish I knew.

That is the certainty I have in life is that I really do not know, I suspect in this life I may never. But what I do know is that the human body is a marvel as is any other species on this Planet. Just think of all we are capable of achieving only in one life time, think about the billions of lifetimes there are, have been, and will be. That is why it is so important not only to take care of our bodies, but of the Planet as well, she is our true Mother.

Before I had left on my adventures around the World I was beginning to get very much out of shape and I was getting concerned. I knew why, I had not been working physically for sometime, I was eating far too much food, and a lot of the wrong kinds of food.

(Apparently I am Human.) Guess what happened? I started to put on weight, get the all to popular beer belly, and generally feeling run down. Even though I was on one of the best Multivitamins on the market.

I had stopped doing my daily push ups, reduced the distance I was walking, if I walked at all on some days. I do not include the usual walking around the home as any form of exercise, unless you count walking up a flight of twenty stairs or more fifty times a day. Well, I was on my way to being fat, lethargic, and feeling horrible. It did not take long, about four months. So there I was 55 years of age and twenty pounds over my ideal weight of about 160lbs. maybe I should take up smoking too.

The one important thing about travelling on a budget, I knew I would be walking plenty. Boy was I right. At this point two and a half months in I have averaged about 6KM per day. I am still doing my push ups, and as always my goal is to do at least my age...55 push ups at least every second day. If I feel energetic, I throw in a couple of sets of ten sit ups.

I am now down to my ideal weight, I feel so much better, and no beer belly. I still indulge every once in a while and have a few, just not every day, and no more than about 3 or 4 at any given time. My diet is better, it is a challenge when you are travelling, I am eating less and try to stick with the fruits and vegetables and not too much meat and the only meat I eat is poultry and seafood as I mentioned earlier. Becoming and staying healthy is certainly a state of mind.

With the World the way it is today, with so many stress's it is more of a challenge than ever. Your attitude will go a long way in either facilitating your long term plans and those of others around you, or can derail a plan and take others with you.

A common goal works well for most people, and working in a group can enlarge the possibilities. There are focus groups, brain storming groups, jogging clubs, and just about anything else you can think of, the secret here is in numbers, generally no less than about five. You will be gleaning off the others in the group as they are also doing the same thing.

By having common goals and a set of flexible rules, most in the group should experience a reasonable amount of success. When it comes to the overall health of a group, consideration must be allowed for in the individual and the unique circumstances surrounding that person. No two people are alike. The main goal for any group or individual should be to replace old habits with new ones that will facilitate the desired outcome. Which is of course a healthier mind and body and planet.

Local gyms, like the **YM/YWCA** be great places to get a start as these gyms will have all of the equipment necessary and trained personnel to help you along. Mind you, gyms are not cheap and there is no point in joining one unless you make the effort to use it at least three times per week.

Often the fact that one has paid money for something will force them into using the facilities. I for a number of years used a local gym and found it very rewarding. However, do not fall into the trap of trying to impress others, or yourself by over extending your abilities, this will generally result in some sort of injury and possibly a long term one. This happened to me and many others I know.

When I help people with an exercise program now, I emphasize the benefits of using light weights with very slow reps. For instance; If you can say bench press 100 pounds comfortably, then try about 25% of that weight and do your reps slowly, count to yourself 30 seconds up, then 30 seconds down and do as many reps as you can.

This will stress the muscle, bone, and ligaments to a higher degree than using a very heavy weight. The difference? Minimal chance of injury to muscle, bone, or ligament. You'll be surprised at how difficult it can be, but safe.

So again some small changes and an attitude change and things start to come together and make for a better life for you, your family and friends, and of course the planet. I will emphasize that the Planet of course is the most important piece to this puzzle. From what we understand, the planet has been here a very long time, and in all likely hood will be here for a very much longer time, we might be talking billions of years here. That would make our lives somewhat inconsequential to the big picture. Maybe not.

This is something we just do not know. So if we do not know what the future holds, doesn't it make sense to live a life of harmony with nature and our own bodies? When we think alike with our surroundings we become closer to what and who we really are. It becomes an intuition kind of existence, one we should trust over many other indicators that have over the centuries proven unreliable.

Trust is a difficult concept for us humans to grasp. But it is one we must, if we are to continue, and to continue in a balanced way with our fellow comrades on this planet. I have often thought that a step back in evolutionary history could solve many of problems, especially our health. I sit here now writing in Portugal. The Mediterranean diet has been hailed as one of the most beneficial diets in the World. I am now experiencing it first hand. Even with the occasional abuse of certain foods such as dairy, sugars, and wheat, I am still overall feeling rather good.

Physically I am doing no more than the locals, which for anyone back home would amount to a serious hike up a large mountain. A lot of walking here, and where I am at, plenty of hills. My body loves the work and appreciates the better food. It may also have something to do with the difference in eating schedules.

Here, breakfast is not too early and for most, the day starts around nine AM. A long break early afternoon where again most will have the large meal for the day with a break afterwards, then finish up the day maybe around six or seven in the evening with a late modest meal. Sometimes even 10 PM for the last meal of the day.

So far it seems to have a relaxing affect on the body. Again, a better attitude towards a balanced lifestyle. I have noticed here in Portugal that many people smoke. From the young to the old, Women and Men. It is hard for me to get used to as back home in Canada we have such strict rules about smoking around others you hardly notice it. Here in Portugal, you can smell it everywhere.

I am aware however that there does not seem to be a direct apparent health issue. Possibly the tobacco is of a different quality and I am guessing with a lower stress level, better diet, more exercise, and more sunshine, (Vitamin D) which they have found to be very important not only for everyone, but especially for smokers. This somehow keeps many from the ravages of smoking.

I have just met a young woman here in Portugal that is the true meaning of a free spirit and has one of the best attitudes I have come across in such a long time. She is not concerned with money, marriage, owning things. She eats a simple yet nutritious diet, gets plenty of low impact exercise, spends a large part of her day outdoors, refuses to have any stress issues, and looks very healthy. She has adopted the attitude of living for the moment. This kind of attitude can only help with any health issues. Any non required stress always takes a toll on the overall health of the body.

True, it can be difficult to reduce or eliminate these stress's, but it is important to make the shift, no matter how small or insignificant it may seem. Just remember, the definition of insanity is doing the same thing over and over, then expecting different results. Change the attitude, a balanced life will follow. It is never too late to make the changes, but one must make them to become a better, and healthier person. It's all in the attitude.

CHAPTER TEN - BEING INFORMED THEN DOING IT.

I hope to this point you are getting at least some useful information that you can apply right away to making changes for the better in your search for great health. Being informed these days is so very easy. The internet is a treasure trove of countless places you can go to get information on almost anything you can think of. It can also steer you in the wrong direction. It seems you have to be well informed even to get useful information from the internet. I often encourage people when they ask me about certain health issues to not only take heed to what I say, but to also find other professionals to talk with and then make an informed decision as to what it is they might want to proceed with.

Everyone is unique, no two people will require the same diet, same physical workout, same medical requirements. This is why it is so important for any individual to really know who they are and how their body works. Just don't take someone's word for it, not even mine. Not even your doctor's. Do the research, be satisfied that you have exhausted every lead and you know without a doubt what it is you're body needs or does not need at any given time.

Everyone should get no less than three opinions from three different qualified health professionals about a potentially serious medical issue which brings on any unusual symptoms. Too many people arbitrarily take information they receive to be the only course of action they should take. They trust their health practitioner, and so they think they should. These days however, in most places around the World Doctors have been educated in primarily one mode of operation. Drug therapy.

Even my own doctor admits to this practice, of training doctors to administer drugs for almost any complaint a patient may have. I am not saying some intervention with certain drug therapy can not be useful, I just find it hard to swallow, (sorry for the pun) that it seems all of a sudden we humans need an assortment of drugs to combat even the simplest of symptoms.

As you now know, there are over 70,000 different man made chemicals on this planet, and most of them end up in our bodies either through drugs, food, or even just the air we breath. I think I have mentioned this enough throughout this book. Many of these drugs never leave our bodies, continuing a life long assault on our health. Patients need to be informed, and unfortunately this task has become the responsibility of the patient. To get the correct information can be even more difficult than one could imagine.

Even with the advent of the internet, most information is directed at people who at some time may purchase a product, and we all know how far sales people will go for a sale. So, not only do you now need a qualified doctor, which is hard to find, but you will also need someone to decipher all of the information you can glean from the internet.

We as patients need to be more aggressive in our requirements when it comes to choosing a doctor. We have to set new standards and stop accepting the poor information we are getting about our health and the health of our family. A good first question to ask a prospective doctor might be where in their class did they graduate. Top, middle, or bottom.

You might just want to know. Not all doctors are in the business to just help, many are in for the money, prestige, ego inflation, power, and so on. When you find a doctor strictly in the business for the sake of the patient, this will be a keeper. Remember, they did take an oath, "**First do no harm**."

The internet again is a place you can go to check out most doctors and their business history. Remember? It is your health, and the health of your family at risk here, you are entitled to the best information, and the best methods to treat any medical issue. It should never come down to money.

Too many people are forced because of our financial system to settle for inferior medical advice and procedures, and are then convinced to start a daily ritual of pill taking that for the most part will do nothing but cause them grief and more medical issues.

I am an avid reader, so getting information seems to be no problem for me. Others, may not have the time, resources, or inclination to do so, that does not mean they are not entitled to the best quality medical care available.

I mentioned earlier that I often venture outside our Canadian medical system, (which is considered to be one of the better ones globally) to find accurate and common sense information. This is an additional cost to me which I find not to be a problem as I know I am getting the best information I can.

Having a health care system such as that in Canada, we should have that kind of information and health care without the extra expense and feel secure in knowing we are getting the best our system has to offer. Unfortunately, money always becomes an issue, and people suffer because of it. Again.

If we as a species are to continue on the path we are on, (which at the moment is to apparently to populate every square inch of this planet). We should also be able to look after the billions of humans we create. Everyone, and for that matter every other species on this planet deserve the quality of life it seems is only reserved for the wealthy. This can only change when the majority of us demand better health care and open and honest education.

Good health, or for that matter great health is not unachievable, it is as I have pointed out in the title "So Simple" As I write this particular chapter, I am still in Portugal. Here I see the contrast that is becoming so commonplace these days. The local Portuguese, that is the older ones, seem so vibrant and healthy. They for the most part are in great shape, many are not on a long list of drugs, and have an active lifestyle into their eighties, nineties, and beyond.

My observation here draws me to the conclusion that the local people get more than their fair share of sunshine, which is the best Vitamin D supplement on the market. Their lifestyle is for the most part stress free, they take a long midday lunch.

I notice also that no one rushes about. They are religious and churches are abundant. The food is for the most part fresh, untampered with, and they celebrate the family. Children and adults alike are together throughout the day. They walk far more than any Canadians or Americans do, and in to late age, many without the use of canes, walkers, or motorized chairs. This is a country where the streets are narrow, the walkways narrow and treacherous, and plenty of hills.

The air in the country is clear, most likely because there are fewer cars and trucks on the road, and the ones that are, use less fuel and run cleaner than most North American vehicles. All of this adds up to a better and healthier lifestyle.

In contrast, when the tourists arrive here in Albufeira, on the coast and a part of the Algarve, you can see how different the lifestyle must be in Northern Europe and the UK. People of similar age are walking with canes, they are overweight, they look sickly and have a difficult time negotiating the narrow walkways and hills. When you see them eat their food at restaurants, it is the greasy fried foods, devoid of most nutrients that got them where they are with their health today.

The obvious lack of sunshine I'm sure plays a large roll in the health or lack of it. Another thing I noticed was that here in Portugal, and I assume in many European states, a large segment of the population smoke cigarettes.

The comparison however is that the local Portuguese seem to fair better with it than those of Canada, North America, or Northern Europe. Again, I believe it to be the sun. Of course the locals do not use sunscreen, and neither should anyone else, especially children. If you can't eat it, don't put it on your skin! Period. People often say, "Then I'll burn if I don't use sunscreen." Get out of the sun after about fifteen to twenty minutes. Most of the beneficial nutrients from the sun enter through your eyes anyway.

The locals here in Portugal don't wear sunglasses or sunscreen, they wear hats and cover up for the most part. The key to getting the right amount of sunshine for ones health is to be moderate, and allow only a small percentage of exposed skin to the sun. Ideally in the morning and late afternoon. This is why the Mediterranean lifestyle works so well and is promoted as one of the best lifestyles anywhere in the World.

So, if you want to get on a program to better your health, adopt the Mediterranean lifestyle as much as you can. If you live in a northern clime, it will be difficult to get enough good sun. You can now get cost effective light therapy that imitates this process, but my guess is, it is still not as good as the real thing.

Fresh organic fruit and vegetables, lots of olive oil, garlic, and onions. Fish, and the occasional glass of good wine, from what I can see, it works just fine, and it is simple. Since I have been in Portugal my health has improved. I walk on average about five kilometres per day, I get plenty of sunshine, without burning, I eat a nutritious balanced diet, drink filtered water, and an occasional glass of red wine. My stress has been reduced to practically nothing, and the hospitality that the locals extend contributes to the mandatory social requirements for ones state of health.

I think if you were to sit down and explain to a local Portuguese person the daily lifestyle of a

North American, they would laugh themselves off their chair. It is not complicated, some of us just tend to like doing things that way. Being informed is crucial these days to knowing what you should and shouldn't do. We can't all live in the Mediterranean, but we can adopt some of the same principles of their lifestyle. We can use new therapies and medications if they have been proven to be beneficial and non harmful.

In order to get the right information one has to know where to go to get it. I will do my best and supply you with places and doctors you can go to for advice. This is for the most part on the internet through online newsletters. you will soon decide for yourself which ones you should pay attention to, and which ones sound a little off the wall. All information is good if you use it to improve your lifestyle. These websites will be posted at the end of the last chapter.

CHAPTER ELEVEN - PERSONAL CARE

When I talk about personal care, I am referring more to what goes into your body, we already know not to put anything on your body unless it is something your body can handle internally. Why do we eat? I often thought how easy it would be to exist on this Planet if we never had to eat food, or drink water. It would be so simple.

There are some species that do not require food intake for as long as two years. These are the kinds of biological systems that make sense on a planet that has a limited supply of resources. We eat simply because our bodies need nutrients to process and continue the strengthening of our cells which in turn repair and strengthen all of our body parts. Again a simple process that we as humans tend to complicate.

With adequate mobility, and rest, the average adult body requires no more than about two thousand calories per day, and between four to six eight ounce glasses of water. There is one group that suggests fewer calories per day. The Life Extension Group. Nineteen hundred calories per day.

The logic behind this is that our bodies could be compared to that of a tree or plant. When a tree or plant is pruned, either through natures way or that of human intervention. The plant becomes stronger and produces more fruit, flowers, or whatever it is the plant manufactures. This is a self defence mechanism.

Our bodies work in somewhat the same manner. Restrict what it is our bodies need, and the result is stronger cells being made to facilitate a perceived threat. Such as starvation. If the fine line can be maintained, the theory is your body will never age, or age very little. Even if this fine line is not maintained, a reduction in calories seems to be beneficial.

I look back at wartime prisoners, especially those that had been imprisoned for many years with sub grade food and unsanitary living conditions. Many, after being released lived on to a somewhat healthy old age compared to their counterparts who threw caution to the wind and ate just about anything they wanted, and a lot of it.

Many cultures have ritual fasting that has been a part of their culture for thousands of years. In part, it was involuntary, but when positive and healthy results were experienced, it was obvious that restriction on a regular basis was good. Think of it like your vehicle, if you have one. You wouldn't think of driving it for a full year without at least changing the oil once or twice. Of course people are sceptical.

Mothers are generally always prompting their children to eat more, not less. Of course this is instinctual for any Mother. My Mother included. Every time though I go on a fast or cleanse, I always feel better, and look better. Just to be clear, a cleanse is not the same as a fast, and both need a strong informational base to accomplish.

The easiest way to experience a true fast is to not eat any food for one day. Make sure you consume some good water, and keep the exertion to a minimum. Those that have disorders that require a certain amount of sugar through proper nutrition should not do this unless under qualified supervision.

It is not difficult, of course your brain will keep telling you to eat some food, especially the bad kind, because that is the kind our brain craves. Just realize though that we do not eat for at least eight to ten hours a day depending on how much sleep you get on any given night, and of course providing you do not have the nasty habit of waking up and going to the refrigerator for late night snacks. This is why they call it Break-fast.

You are breaking the fast from the night before. We all know what happens when you do not have this break. We tend to put on the pounds. Now let's talk about an affliction that is becoming ever increasing, the results from constant eating of poor grade foods, and virtually no movement.

Obesity, extreme obesity. This is the result of continually eating far too many calories while doing virtually no movement. There are many

175

people that have this affliction. They cannot stop eating. Between 10,000 and 30,000 calories per day, and the food is of poor quality. Some of these people can reach a body weight of over a 1,000 pounds!

They can only be moved in many cases by the removal of entire walls. The majority of these people are between 400 and 600 pounds. This is a brain problem more than anything else. That is why it is important to listen to the stomach and understand its signals, and not the brain. In most cases the brain is secondary to your digestive system. Hence, "That gut feeling." one gets.

The most common way to reverse this affliction is to reduce the size of the stomach, make it so small that one is feeling full after only consuming one or two mouthfuls of food. This can work temporarily, but like I said, the brain is the problem and it will find a way. What a lot of people do in this predicament is to eat continuously again putting on far too much fat. The only way, and the only safe way is to re-train the brain and eat properly and move.

When people get to this point in their disease, your brain has come to the conclusion that you are dying. Only for the lack of movement. When a person weighs more than 600 pounds, they do not move very much and this signals to the brain that death will come sooner than later. The body goes into a defence mode. Like I said earlier, when your body does this on a short fast, it can be good for the body, but when one is extremely obese and continues to eat constantly without movement, even though you have plenty of food, the brain is getting a much different message. It will still think you are starving and that is why these people continue to eat. For one thing, the food is readily available, if it was not, these people would have to move themselves to get it, or starve.

If you are not ready for fasts, or cleanses, (Which are similar to fasts, but incorporate some amount of nutrition, either through juices, certain light foods, or soups) then a good rule of thumb for the average adult would be to consume between 1900 to 2500 calories per day depending on exertion levels.

These calories of course should be of the highest

quality one can obtain. Organic fruits and vegetables, organic fish, poultry, beef, pork, and any other meats. (I'll get into meats in a minute) a few handfuls of quality nuts and seeds, and good whole grains.

The use of the word organic can be misleading, especially these days as there are so many companies out there trying to get your money. Pretty much if the food is packaged, it is not top quality. That is why most nutritionists will always say, stay away from the middle isles of the supermarket.

It is important to know where your food is coming from. This was not an issue one hundred years ago, even fifty years ago in most places. If not from your garden, farm, or fish boat, then know who's it is from.

Many people these days eat far too much red meat, the wrong kind, I believe humans are at least for now required in some way to ingest a small amount of meat per week. One has to remember we evolved from a hunter gatherer society and you cannot change something like this overnight. In biological terms overnight could be 100,000 years. I am not saying one can't be strictly vegetarian, there are many that are, it just takes a lot more work and research. One day we may very well thrive only on a vegetarian diet. We as a species are continually changing.

The meat most people consume has been completely altered from its natural state. Just visit a feed lot, chicken barn, hog barn, turkey barn, fish pen, and the list goes on. Most animal products have been genetically modified, grown with the addition of drugs, antibiotics, colourings, steroids, growth hormones, elevated sodium injection, plastics, animal feces, tainted blood, and I am sure this list goes on as well.

Know where your meat comes from and make sure it is natural, or at least as natural as one can get these days. If the cow you bought had a name, it is likely better meat. When you see a cow, sheep, pig, or any other two or four legged animal running free and eating what it naturally wants to eat, then you know you will be getting a better quality meat than that of a feed lot prisoner.

Don't think your seafood is any safer. With the continuous practice of over fishing, dumping of raw sewage and garbage into our oceans, the offshore drilling for oil and natural gas, and the proliferation of fish farming, it is a wonder we have any life in our oceans at all. Seafood itself if it is of good quality, is good for us as a good source of vitamins and minerals. As pointed out previously, that, is getting harder to find.

On the topic of fish farming, it has been suggested that a fish from a farm as opposed to a wild fish is almost completely opposite in beneficial nutrients. A wild, natural fish is generally full of omega 3's, a fatty acid very beneficial to us humans and many other species.

The farmed fish however have a reverse and have far less omega 3 fatty acids. This is due mainly to their feed, which is a manufactured pellet that does not resemble in any way what a fish would eat in the wild.

Instead of being heart healthy for us, it becomes the opposite, bad for our hearts in the form of bad cholesterol. To make things worse, colourings are used to make the fish look like the fish we are used to eating. These practises have to stop if we are to ever get back on track with a balance and nutritious diet.

The fat is different, the essential oils are different, the entire fish has for the most part been genetically modified. Stay clear of farm raised fish. Even the wild species of large fish, such as Tuna, Shark, and Marlin are now known to have unacceptable levels of mercury which has been linked to the over use of fossil fuels globally.

We now know what horrible effects Mercury can have on a human. If one has trouble obtaining good food, which most do in North America and other so called advanced countries, then how do you obtain the nutrients your body requires on a daily basis?

Multivitamins. There, I said it. Many people turn their nose up at this quite new phenomena. There have been many scams, thousands of products lining the shelves of millions of pharmacies, supermarkets, and health food stores, and a general mistrust of what it is these products are supposed to accomplish. I agree. In part.

Most nutritional supplements are inferior and some are even dangerous. Again it is important to know where something is coming from especially if you are ingesting it, or feeding it to your children. I suggest reading the "**Comparative Guide to Nutritional Supplements**"

Thirty or forty years ago, I would have said, "Vitamin supplements? I'll get it from my food thank you." But not today. The results are in, and most, if not all food we consume is deficient in a multitude of nutrients that our bodies require every day. The soils have been depleted of nutrients, the sun has to filter through smog encased cities, water used to irrigate the fields is polluted, and the chemicals used to replace what nature did so well are deadly.

Without a good multivitamin our bodies don't stand a chance. The operative word here is "Good'. Again one has to do their due diligence in finding a good quality vitamin. Plenty of reading, researching a company that proclaims a miraculous side affect, knowing where and how raw ingredients are processed, independent scientific studies done on the products. Again, overwhelming. I will at the end of the book give you resources as to which company has the best vitamins and body products available.

If we are unsure as to whether or not we are getting sufficient quality nutrients in our daily food, which we are most certainly not, unless you are personally producing the food and doing the testing, then I think it important to supplement with some that have been proven to be not only necessary in our diets, but crucial to our long term health, and of course those that have gone through the scrutiny of not only Government agencies, but independent as well.

It is far from perfect, but supplementation is now a certain requirement if we are to become as healthy as we can. With the simple fact that vitamins are in a capsule or pill form makes it somewhat foreign to our digestive systems. Whole foods if they are of good quality are far superior. Don't exclude a multivitamin regime if you know the company to have very high standards in efficacy, regular testing, natural organic ingredients, and have adopted a planet friendly way of production. Until we can get our planet back to what it once was, supplementation will be here to stay.

CHAPTER TWELVE - BIG BUSINESS, THE NEW DRUG LORDS

FDA. Ring a bell. The **Federal Drug Administration**. Not a very well received branch of the US Government these days. This organization is supposed to be looking out for our welfare, you, the individual. Canada has a similar agency, the Canadian Food and Drug Agency and I am sure most countries have something similar.

It should be obvious to anyone that with all of the recalls on both sides of the border between Canada and the US of a wide variety of not only food products, but a number of medications as well, these Government watchdogs are not doing their job. It comes down to you, you cannot expect someone else to do what is best for you when money in most instances is the motivating factor.

When I was growing up as a young teenager in the late sixties, recreational drugs were becoming very popular. The pressure from ones peers to experiment with some of these drugs was enormous. By the time I was in my late twenties, I had sworn off any of these drugs permanently. It wasn't as bad back then for drug dealers to hound you and try to get you hooked on a drug. It was their lively hood, their income was dependent on people becoming life long customers. Even though that life would be considerably shortened.

The authorities came down hard, and did their best to eliminate the dealers, and the drugs, but alas, it was just too large a business and of course newer and harsher drugs came along. I remember parents, adults in positions of authority telling us kids the dangers of drug use, and how it would destroy our lives, physically and mentally. Over the years a number of my friends succumbed to the ravages of these drugs and are not here with us anymore because of it.

Things haven't changed much in more than thirty years. The recreational drugs are still out there, and illegal, and causing more problems than ever. But there is a new kid on the block, a new line of drugs, drugs that work on the same principle as the older ones.

These new drugs are called prescription medications. In fact even one of the old ones that is still for the most part illegal in most countries is now available for prescription for a multitude of ailments. **Medical Marijuana**.

Monsanto, a name that should send chills up your spine when ever it is mentioned. This is one of the large drug companies that is determined to change nature. As you probably are already aware, Monsanto genetically modifies crop seeds to have virtually total control over the production of certain kinds of crops. Eventually of course, this can only have detrimental affects on a multitude of similar crops, and many others that do not share any similarities at all.

I recently viewed a video where Bill gates was presenting a speech to Monsanto executives about the benefits of genetically modifying mosquito's for the purpose of warding off the deadly disease Malaria. How this is supposed to work, or even if it could, it is plain and simple, just not right.

186

I am not saying at some point we humans might be able to work in conjunction with nature and produce beneficial species that can work with nature, not just now. Every time we tinker with nature and let it loose without the extensive and necessary testing, we set ourselves up for some disaster down the road all for the sake of money.

The list of other prescription drugs is endless. I won't go into them here, it would take up too much space, too much time. All you need to do is go to your doctor with any complaint, and voila! Just take this pill twice a day for the rest of your life. If patients ever took the time to read the label on the bottle, it might scare them enough to look elsewhere for a more natural way to eliminate their medical problem.

Don't get me wrong here. I believe certain medications in acute situations can be beneficial and help the patient get on the right track, but not long term. That can only create more problems. Our bodies are designed to do all of the repairs necessary. Introducing foreign substances will only confuse the primary system of dealing with adverse health challenges, and restrict the beneficial properties that this system is designed to perform.

One should always look for alternative ways to alleviate symptoms. In most cases their are natural and non invasive ways to deal with the health issue at hand. When I had my initial consultation with my doctor I of course asked many questions. He himself said that much of his training throughout the years was in drug therapy. Drug companies stand to lose billions of dollars if people just went back to a simple and natural way of living life.

The big drug companies will continue to expand, and are possibly even moving in the direction of food products to get us dependent on their products. When ever your doctor is quick to prescribe some drug to you, take some time to do a little investigation on that particular drug and check to see if there is a healthier alternative. There usually is, and many times it is far more cost effective as well.

With the many thousands of drugs on the market it is becoming more difficult to avoid them, especially now that many of these same drugs are showing up in all kinds of places like our drinking water, some food products, and of course the standard bombardment of inoculations when one is young.

There may come a time in the near future when it will be mandatory to have vaccinations and other treatments. We can only hope this does not happen. We as a species need to get back to what nature provides for us, our bodies were
designed to deal with almost anything that can happen, if we would just leave the process alone to its own methods.

Any man-made substance has no place in our biological system. Our bodies do not have the capabilities to deal with such synthetic substances. many times these chemicals and compounds are stored in the body because they cannot be eliminated or used for any beneficial purpose within our bodies. It is up to us to do our own research and look for safer and natural alternatives, they exist, and have so for thousands of years.

Monsanto, a name that should send chills up your spine when ever it is mentioned. This is one of the large drug companies that is determined to change nature. As you probably are already aware, Monsanto genetically modifies crop seeds to have virtually total control over the production of certain kinds of crops. Eventually of course, this can only have detrimental affects on a multitude of similar crops, and many others that do not share any similarities at all.

I recently viewed a video where Bill gates was presenting a speech to Monsanto executives about the benefits of genetically modifying mosquito's for the purpose of warding off the deadly disease Malaria. How this is supposed to work, or even if it could, it is plain and simple, just not right.

I am not saying at some point we humans might be able to work in conjunction with nature and produce beneficial species that can work with nature, not just now. Every time we tinker with nature and let it loose without the extensive and necessary testing, we set ourselves up for some disaster down the road all for the sake of money.

It is just that there is no profit in simple and natural methods. Greed is the real disease. When you travel around the World and experience different lifestyles you begin to understand that the ones with less have better health and live longer. They have to move more, as in walking, they work hard, but also rest and relax more.

Stress is almost non existent. Family life is just that..family. It is the people with more money that have more problems, especially with their health, you can see it everywhere. Life was meant to be simple, not complicated.

If we continue to allow our Governments to work hand in hand with these large corporations and continue to let them put dangerous drugs on the market before extensive and conclusive testing has been done, we will surely be in a sorry state in the near future. We are already allowing children to be given drugs for such things as depression, diabetes, and ADHD, which I think is a totally made up diagnosis. The large drug companies operate no differently than the drug dealers on the street I was familiar with so many years ago.

The easiest way to turn this around, is to refuse the drugs in the first place. One hundred years ago there were virtually no drugs, and we still for the most part managed to live a healthy life. You say, "But John, drugs have eliminated some of our worst disease's."

My response is that if left to nature, they would have been eliminated as well. In any case, some are now returning. We should just lay down the weapons and accept defeat when it comes to trying to control the environment. There is no logic in it, and certainly nothing positive will come of it. It is only being done for the greed and power of a few.

CHAPTER THIRTEEN - WHAT

ABOUT THE YOUNG?

It is somewhat easy to talk about all that goes on with our health these days as a middle aged man. I have lived long enough to understand some things, and make changes for myself for the better, but what about the young?

What kind of a World will they have to exist in? When a young child today is given far too many vaccinations, over the counter remedies for a multitude of common childhood ailments, and given sub-grade food, if you can even call some of it food. Two to three generations ago most people lived simple and productive lives with reasonably good diets of natural foods not yet tampered with by humans.

Children today do not stand a chance. And if the large drug companies have their way, every single human will have to be on some kind of drug. I suspect in the future mainly as a control mechanism. We will become like sheep, walking through the largest garbage dump in the universe.

As I stated earlier in the book, many people at the top of large corrupt corporations are sociopaths. They have no feelings and could care less about anything other than power over almost everything.

I was born into a generation where food production was just starting to use harmful chemicals on a mass scale to mimic the natural cycle of nature. Providing man-mad chemicals to plants and animals started the never ending cycle of poor health, then the use of inferior drugs to try and correct these inefficiencies. Today, organic farmers will tell you that their farming practises are more cost effective, and more profitable than the use of synthetic fertilizers used by large corporate farms.

Now that I know how food production is done, especially here in North America, I have made changes to my lifestyle to accommodate these harmful methods of food production. The young today do not have that option as their bodies are already toxic due to the continual ingestion of harmful drugs. And even through their Mother when in her womb.

At certain times throughout the year I take

measures to help flush out harmful chemicals from my body by doing cleanses and mini-fasts. I mentioned this earlier in the book and highly recommend it as a way of getting your body back, or at least close to it, normal.

Most of the young people today do not understand how important it is to maintain a balance within their bodies. To fight off disease and other deficiencies, a body must have the right tools to work with, mainly nutrient rich foods, and quality drinking water.

Many of these harmful chemicals will also find their way into our bodies through the air that we breath. I read an article some years ago stating that the actual percentage of oxygen in our atmosphere had diminished by about 25% over the past 100,000 years. Whether that is due to a natural process, or one that has been brought on by over industrialization is anyone's guess. The fact remains, that even without all of the airborne pollutants, we, and many other species are breathing in a different oxygen than years ago.

People who live in, or close to large cities have a higher incidence of cardio related illness. It has become difficult to find places where the air is clear and good for you. Automobiles are the largest culprit, and with China and India coming on board with their economic stimulus, there will be considerably more vehicles vying for a spot on our already congested roadways.

There is new technology to reduce the problems inherent with fossil fuel driven vehicles, but it seems to be coming on line to slowly to turn around the problems our oil addicted society has produced. There are air driven cars, solar driven cars, electric cars, hydrogen powered cars, and my guess is we will eventually go back in time and give the steam driven car another go. Until we make some very major fundamental shifts in the way we live, our health and that of the planet and other species will continue to suffer.

We see it more and more that the young are starting to get the picture and protest the status quo. It will be vitally important that we, an older generation listen and take up the fight along with them to not only protect our planet, but to re-instate the homoeostasis of our fragile environment. Not just for us humans, but all species. Without this, our planet will rebel and do for us what we should have been doing all along. Your children, grandchildren, and possibly your great grandchildren deserve a better future. The only way they will be able to achieve that is if they can be healthy along with a healthy planet.

What can you do to help? Every chance you get, do your best to explain to the young what it is we have done to this beautiful planet, and what is needed to put it back on the right track. Come back to basics. Keep it simple.

There are approximately seven billion humans on this planet, according to some experts that is about six billion too many for the available resources here on our planet, and remember, we have to share these resources with many other species. Our planet is the most important component of the equation. We need to be able to produce good quality food, water, air, for a few, and keep this planet clean for future generations of all species.

By being of sound mind and body we can make better choices because our minds are not cluttered with too many things, and is a healthy mind because it was given all of the right nutrients so it can grow strong, same with the rest of our body, it all works as one smooth operating machine.

No one part is separate from another. With more

and more people returning to traditional farming methods, the message is slowly getting out. With more and more people becoming sick because of past, and present manufacturing and food processing, it has become clear that what we have been doing to our most important resource, food. Not only for the consumption of humans..but all living species.

I take responsibility for damaging our fragile environment, and anyone that is alive today is also. Once we admit to our mistakes, we can begin anew and start to repair the damage we have done. The generations yet to come must know that we are human, and we have the capacity to make mistakes. I think we are even far beyond that and can turn this planet around and create the garden of Eden we have heard about.

We have to break old habits and start the clean up process, if the younger ones see us taking on this monumental challenge, they will surely pitch in and give a helping hand. It starts with you becoming healthy through doing the right things. This in turn shows the way for others. Only healthy people can make the right choices, only healthy children can guarantee any future at all for future generations of humans, and other species we share this planet with.

CHAPTER FOURTEEN - THE EXTENDED FORECAST

What do I see for the future? I do not have a crystal ball, I cannot see into the future, I can only hope. If I see change for the better, then I see hope for the future. As I stated in the previous chapter, we all have to buckle down and do what is right. It may be to late for some of us, but we can start the process for making a cleaner and healthier planet for all in the future.

I would like to extend to you the reader a challenge. To become first of all a healthier human being. Do everything in your power to put into, and onto your body only those things that are of nature. Possibly in the future humankind might be able to re-create certain things in nature, but for now we have not done a very good job. Money always seems to get in the way. A simple lifestyle should be the goal.

Keep the unnecessary at bay. Technology is a fantastic tool, and I am sure it will be even more fantastic in the future. But we need to control it and not the other way round. Too many people are tied to their cell phones, iPod, laptops, computers, TV's and so on. They are all great, of course I use them myself. but I do not lose sight of what is really important here, connecting not to our electronic devices, but to our nature, our Planet we call home.

The challenge may appear to be insurmountable, but taken a step at a time can be overcome. Start today with one small, simple step. Instead of a doughnut for coffee break, have a carrot, or an apple. Certified Organic of course.

This one small step will influence your shopping patterns, which will influence some of those around you, and so on. Do not let big business push you around, it is supposed to be the other way round. Big business, big Government, is in your control, always has been. If we are to become healthier humans, we need to let those that produce our food and other products know, we are ready for a change. If not for ourselves, at least our children and theirs.

We need to take the blinders off and take a real good look around, see what it is we have created, not to just look at the nice things, but the ugly as well. We can only sweep the dirt under the carpet for so long, eventually we all will have to deal with it. Even those that are doing what's right.

If you are at home right now, it is a nice day, you are thinking about what to get for dinner, and you live within a kilometre or two of a good supermarket. Get the family together and a few cloth shopping bags and all of you walk to the supermarket, walk in and go right to the produce section, find the certified organic produce and get some wholesome good food for you and your family. Sure it will cost you more, but when everyone is buying only the good stuff the prices will fall. It is actually cheaper to produce organic produce than the chemically laden stuff so many of us have been forced to buy.

The walk was good for you, the conversation with the family was good for you, and the food you purchased will be good for you. This is how it used to be done, this is how it is still done in many countries, and this is how it must be done, and when you get home, get the family together to cook. Not in a microwave, but a real oven. Feel the warmth, smell the aromas, this is what food consumption is all about. It is a spiritual event. You're body, you're health
depend on it.

Our planet is going through some major growing pains. There is plenty of unrest, military turmoil, environmental issues, more and more political unrest, and of course...the list continues to grow. The old saying comes to mind; "**It is always darkest just before the day dawneth.**" *Thomas Fuller.*

I truly believe we will come out the other end a better species and will use what we have learned to make this Planet what it once was and better. It will certainly not be an easy task, and nor should it be. The harder a challenge, the better the results. If you and as many people as you can influence to just take a few small steps in the right direction just think about how much better things will be. Cleaner air, cleaner water, actual real food, and many Eco-systems returning to their original diversity.

We as a species must put aside petty little differences, and acknowledge the importance of repairing, and maintaining this very special planet. There are many doomsayers out there, and sometimes even I sound much like it might be hopeless.

But that here is the operative word..HOPE. And as

long as we have that, anything is possible. So when you look in the mirror tomorrow morning and see a not to healthy human being, just remember that the formula is simple, and a small step in the right direction can, and will bring with it a small success in the right direction.

I know in my heart that many thousands of years from now, humans will look back at this time and wonder why we allowed such a dangerous disease to infect nearly every human on the planet, that disease is the disease of greed and power.

That brings to mind another resource you might want to watch, a documentary called **"The Age of Stupid"** are the only two things that put us humans in the so very unhealthy situation we are in today. Take money and Power out of the equation and balance will be achieved.

Many of us find that difficult to comprehend as we have all been trained from a young age to follow the lead of people whose only goal in life is to accumulate wealth and power at any cost, just take a look at our environment, it is in a shambles, and the only way to fix it is to make changes today, no matter how small they may be.

We can have everything we want in life, the tasty treats, the wonderful books, movies, art, and music. The fun, laughter, and especially a long and healthy life. We just have to stand up and demand that we go back to a simple process and only do what it is we want to do if, and only if, it is in harmony with our planet and its Eco-system. I will leave you with this thought, and I trust you will make better decisions tomorrow while standing in front of that mirror.

"All good is not lost, it is only hidden for now by the collective ignorance of a misguided, and frightened leadership."

"May you're God stand beside you and guide you along the right path to happiness and health."

"So Simple, Who Knew?"

John P. Gibson

RESOURCES

Here is some information that may, or may not be of help to you. After doing your due diligence, you can make an educated decision.

Doctors I recommend reading up on through newsletters or information gathered on the internet.

Dr. Myron Wentz USANA Health Sciences

"Comparative Guide to Nutritional Supplements" Dr. Lyle MacWilliam

Dr. John Cline - Specializes in Chelation Therapy. Has a clinic in Nanaimo, BC Canada. Website address:
www.clinemedical.com

Dr. Douglas www.realhealthnews.com

Dr. Williams www.davidwilliams.com

Dr. Yam A Natureopathic clinic in Victoria, BC Canada

Dr. Shelton "Food Combining Made Easy" Book

Dr. Henry Lodge and Chris Crowley The book "Younger Next
Year" www.youngernextyear.com

Dr. Whitaker www.julianwhitaker.com

Nutrition and Healing Newsletter www.healthiernews.com

Consumer Labs Newsletter www.consumerlab.com

Health Sciences Institute HSI Newsletter www.healthsciencesinstitute.co.uk

Water Filters and Distillers www.waterwise.com www.steripen.com

Books and Movies

"Mad Cowboy" Book by Howard Lyman www.madcowboy.com

"Detoxify or Die" Book by Sherry A. Rogers

"WALL-E" Animated movie

"Idiocracy" Movie

"The Age of Stupid" Documentary

Both "**WALLEE**"and "**Idiocracy**" **though** being entertainment type movies have an underlying message worth noting.